Using Qualitative Metho
Determinants of Health Research

This book provides researchers, faculty, and students with a comprehensive resource for applying qualitative methods in Social Determinants of Health (SDOH) research among underrepresented communities.

Addressing a significant gap in existing literature, this book extends beyond traditional qualitative texts by offering targeted instruction on utilizing these methods to explore social, cultural, environmental, and political factors that shape health inequities. It is an extension of texts that define qualitative research, distinguish qualitative from quantitative research, and provide instruction or guidance on ways to implement, analyze, and evaluate this methodology in populations experiencing illness events. Key features include practical guidance on conducting qualitative research throughout the entire study process—from planning and data collection to analysis and dissemination. The author draws on over 20 years of experience, integrating real-world examples that illustrate the effective use of qualitative methods in diverse contexts.

Ideal for researchers and faculty in nursing, public health, medicine, theology, and divinity, it serves as a resource for emerging and experienced scholars who may be initiating new projects on SDOH, integrating SDOH into existing research, and/or adapting measures or interventions for cultural relevance among underrepresented communities. It is also a vital resource for those teaching and mentoring students in rigorous and innovative SDOH research.

Jill B. Hamilton, PhD, MRPL, RN is a tenured Professor at the Nell Hodgson Woodruff School of Nursing and Affiliate Professor at Candler School of Theology at Emory University in Atlanta, Georgia, USA. Dr. Hamilton earned a BSN, MSN, and PhD in nursing from the University of North Carolina at Chapel Hill, a BS in Accounting from North Carolina Central University, and completed postdoctoral training in the nursing care of older adults at the Oregon Health & Science University.

Using Qualitative Methods for Social Determinants of Health Research

Exploring Health Inequities

Jill B. Hamilton

Routledge
Taylor & Francis Group
LONDON AND NEW YORK

Designed cover image: Jill B. Hamilton (photo of the home of Leroy and Georgia Hamilton taken by Jerome C. Martin)

First published 2026
by Routledge
4 Park Square, Milton Park, Abingdon, Oxon OX14 4RN

and by Routledge
605 Third Avenue, New York, NY 10158

Routledge is an imprint of the Taylor & Francis Group, an informa business

For Product Safety Concerns and Information please contact our EU representative GPSR@taylorandfrancis.com. Taylor & Francis Verlag GmbH, Kaufingerstraße 24, 80331 München, Germany.

British Library Cataloguing-in-Publication Data
A catalogue record for this book is available from the British Library

ISBN: 9781032984889 (hbk)
ISBN: 9781032984865 (pbk)
ISBN: 9781003598916 (ebk)

DOI: 10.4324/9781003598916

Typeset in Optima
by KnowledgeWorks Global Ltd.

Contents

Acknowledgements

This book is designed to be a resource for researchers, faculty, and pre- and postdoctoral students desiring a greater understanding of how qualitative methods might be useful for SDOH research with underrepresented communities. I am grateful for the clinicians, community partners, and mentees who either contributed to the research used as exemplars in this text or encouraged me to pursue this project.

I would like to acknowledge with gratitude, the support from Nakia C. Best and Autherine Abiri for their continual support throughout this project. I am also grateful to Kimberly Hannon and Qingyang Hu for their editorial assistance.

Preface

Nearly 30 years ago, as a doctoral student, I began my program of research focused on social determinants of health using qualitative methods. I had taken the one basic qualitative methods course offered at that time and purchased a stack of qualitative methods books. As a conscientious doctoral student, I was eager to conduct my first qualitative study on a topic with which I was extremely passionate. I read that stack of qualitative methods books looking for instructions on how to begin my study, how to access communities of color, and how to recruit appropriate participants. I was seeking answers to the questions that would provide the information necessary to begin my research and an understanding on how to analyze the stories from the transcripts I would collect.

I vividly remember approaching one of my doctoral faculty saying, "I am not able to find any books to help me know what questions to ask" and being told, "It's there you just need to look harder." Well, I did find examples of interview questions, but none were appropriate for my specific population or my specific research question. Looking back, I made a lot of mistakes during those early years and learned a lot in the process. I would now like to share what I have learned with the next generation of community-engaged, qualitative researchers examining social influences on stages of wellness and illness.

This book, *Using Qualitative Research Methods for SDOH Research* is written for scholars who may have taken an introductory course in qualitative methods where they were taught the essentials, but still need guidance in the practical application of qualitative methods during the start-up phases of their research; particularly, as they interact with participants from underrepresented communities. Specifically, this book provides content on the practical application of qualitative methods during the planning phases of a qualitative study when making decisions related to sampling strategies, data collection and analysis, and dissemination in peer-reviewed journals.

1 Engaging Community in Research Design, Implementation, Evaluation, and Dissemination

Community-engaged research is generally recognized as an approach to scholarly activities where academic scholars or healthcare systems form collaborative relationships with members of a target population, community organizations, or community stakeholder groups who are equal partners throughout the research process. Scholars have further described this collaboration as one built on trusting and shared decision-making processes that are bidirectional and result in research projects. These processes are further described as those that exist among individuals or groups who are affiliated by common issues or problems affecting the well-being of a patient or community population. In this chapter, I briefly introduce ways to engage the community in the research process using qualitative methods. These strategies are discussed in greater detail with exemplars throughout this book.

Engaging Community in Research Design

Over the years, my program of research has been enriched tremendously from lessons learned while conducting community-engaged qualitative research. Rather than examinations of relationships among variables or associations of one or more variables on outcome variables, research questions in qualitative research focus on understanding why relationships exist (or not), why outcomes exist (or not), or why relationships or outcomes exist under certain situations or among populations or subpopulations.

One way that I have engaged the community in the research process using qualitative methods is to ensure the inclusion of their voice in the identification of problems or research questions. This ensures that the research project is not only relevant but important to the community. During the early phases of my doctoral research, I was interested in the topic of social support among African American cancer patients. At that time, nearly 30 years ago, the three published studies on this topic suggested that African Americans lacked social support during the diagnosis and treatment for cancer. This negative perception of African Americans lacking social support during a life-threatening illness was generally the result of a failure to include the voice of this population in prevailing conceptualizations of this topic. I was committed to changing that predominantly negative narrative to one whereby the strengths and weaknesses were represented in the scientific literature.

Similar to the identification of problems, qualitative methods in community-engaged research help to structure appropriate research questions. Although research questions in qualitative research are designed to explore meanings, experiences, insights, and/or perspectives of individuals or populations of interest, oftentimes research questions are

DOI: 10.4324/9781003598916-1

derived from gaps in the literature from studies conducted among scientists who have had little to no interactions with members of the target population. As a result, these research questions may address a gap in the literature, but that gap lacks the context necessary to capture the broader needs of the community.

As an emerging scholar during my doctoral studies, the findings that African American cancer patients lacked social support were disturbing and not at all consistent with my experience with this patient population. It is important for scientists to realize that comparisons of various aspects of the African American lived experiences to those of non-Hispanic whites without consideration for cultural differences are likely to result in negative evaluations, misinformation, and stereotypes (Collins, 1991; Gamble, 1993). Research is necessary to counter representations of minority populations as deviant and pathological. The research to identify problems and issues of relevance and importance needs to be community based, using rigorous qualitative methods. In my dissertation research, the findings from a qualitative study suggested that African Americans conceptualized, experienced, and engaged in social support interactions differently than those portrayed in the literature but had differing perceptions of individuals engaged in supportive relationships. For example, among African American cancer patients, the emotional support of expressions of love and caring included the presence of others, sharing material resources, encouraging words, and being made to feel needed. Instrumental support extended beyond current conceptualizations linked to monetary gifts. Rather, this support included prayers, assistance to maintain social roles in the community, assistance to remain in the home during illness, and assistance to engage in religious practices or rituals. Informational support extended beyond the advice and information on what to expect during illness. Instead, conceptualizations of informational support included support to validate and help them understand the information received from healthcare providers, and to get healthcare information in a language easily understood.

A second way to engage the community in the research process using qualitative methods is through the identification of appropriate study designs in subsequent quantitative studies. While qualitative studies may open our eyes to topics that need further exploration through qualitative methods, they may also help inform quantitative analyses. My earlier qualitative study led to the development of a culturally relevant measure of social support and an explanatory study to examine hypothesized associations of social support to established outcome measures of quality of life and relationship well-being. Although this early dissertation research identified the strengths of social support and relationships to positive health outcomes, an additional research question was about those situations that were perceived as negative and stressful among networks of family, friends, co-workers, and faith communities. I was especially interested in African Americans' perceptions of cancer stigma, perceptions of illness-related burdens, and ways in which these survivors accessed social support when support from traditional sources was lacking.

A third way to engage the community in the research process using qualitative methods is through the identification of populations most likely to benefit from the research through clearly articulated sampling criteria (i.e., inclusion and exclusion criteria). Inadequate attention to this step in the research process is likely to result in unsuccessful efforts in recruitment, low enrollment, low participant retention rates, and ultimately lacking in information-rich cases. Initially, inclusion and exclusion criteria may be vaguely stated given the nature of uncharted programs of research. However, during interactions with participants and open-ended interviews, researchers are likely to obtain information that enables them to refine, revise, or focus inclusion and exclusion criteria to more accurately enroll participants likely to provide information-rich cases. During the course of open-ended interviews to understand perceptions of social support among African American cancer survivors, I learned that early stage or surgical-treatment-only cancer patients were not likely to experience disruptions in their sources and types of social support. As a result, the interviews were extremely brief and did not produce information-rich cases. In subsequent studies, I made sure to have surgery-only patients in my exclusion criteria. However, I would not have made this adjustment had I not used qualitative methods in my research.

A fourth way to engage the community in the research process using qualitative methods is through the identification of appropriate data collection methods. Data from my dissertation research strongly supported the need for a culturally relevant measure of social support. Using data from in-depth interviews with these African American cancer survivors, we developed the Ways of Helping Questionnaire (WHQ) to capture their unique coping strategies. In this new measure of social support, items were written from in-depth interviews that represented categories of social support used among older African American cancer patients that were limited or absent in existing measures. In future studies, this measure could be used to conduct individualized assessments of older African American survivors' social support needs in future descriptive, explanatory, and intervention studies.

Qualitative research is beneficial not only to the development of new measures but it also informs other aspects of data collection. Through interactions with the target population, I learned information that would ultimately ensure information-rich cases in future qualitative studies but also information to ensure success with future efforts to recruit, enroll, and minimize subject dropouts in quantitative research studies. For example, during the course of conducting qualitative research, investigators might learn the most appropriate times and places to conduct interviews, the most appropriate strategies for completion of surveys, and whether content on the topic is best discussed in one on one or focus group settings.

Community Engagement in Community Programs and Interventions

Qualitative research conducted prior to the design and implementation of a community program or intervention would allow a scientist to ask: What are the strengths and weaknesses of communities that are likely to positively or adversely affect implementation? During interactions with community stakeholders, I frequently hear stories of researchers making requests for assistance with the recruitment of participants to complete surveys or implement programs from funded research without input from the community. Although these programs may offer the community needed resources, the surveys and/or programs are frequently not relevant or responsive to the community's needs. The failure to include the community at the outset of the research unfortunately results in missed opportunities for all parties. The scientist does not obtain the data necessary to make change or the program is not implemented as planned.

In the design of community programs and interventions, stakeholders or members of the target population are not only the experts on issues or problems in their communities but also expert consultants. As expert consultants in the design and implementation of community programs and interventions, these individuals can inform the scientist on the specific advice and resources needed to implement programs. These resources may include information or opinions that bring about a greater understanding or insight into context surrounding the issue or problem. This insight might include information or background about social determinants influencing the problem that would ensure the success of the program or intervention. Expert consultants can inform or advise on the strengths and challenges within communities that are likely to positively or negatively influence the implementation of programs or interventions.

Given a consideration of the strengths of faith-based institutions as the central organization in the African American community, a program developed to address safe housing, healthy foods, crime, and violence in communities will likely be more successful if conducted in collaboration with faith-based institutions. Faith-based institutions have a long history of supporting African American communities. Congregants of faith-based institutions in the African American community have traditionally engaged in activities of contributing their time, services, and money directly to addressing health and social problems that disproportionately affect the larger African American community (Billingsley, 1992; Hill, 1997).

Similarly, researchers who do not listen to the community may develop a lack of consideration of the challenges that might negatively influence the implementation of a community program or intervention. For example, the same programs developed to address safe housing, healthy foods, crime, and violence will likely not be successful without knowledge of the existing social resources of a community. These resources might include a consideration of jobs, income, and education of the community residents and financial resources available to a community's faith-based institutions.

Qualitative research is also useful in determining the appropriate dosing of community programs or interventions. This dosing might include a consideration for the length of the program or intervention, the identification of key players responsible for the delivery of the program or intervention, or whether the program or intervention should be single or multifaceted. An example of a community program or intervention that may benefit from this type of bundling would be one to address access to health care. While the primary intervention would be the provision of transportation and assistance with local housing during treatment, the intervention is likely to be stronger if a component for social support and the influence of social norms on certain illnesses were included. A qualitative aim would enhance the scientist's knowledge of any cultural norms that might strengthen or weaken the dosing of any community programs or interventions.

Evaluation of Programs and Interventions Implemented in Communities

Qualitative research is invaluable in the evaluation of ways community programs or interventions are implemented in the real world. Scientists may use qualitative methods to understand the usability and acceptability of the program or intervention. This exploration might include, for example, the clarity, persuasiveness, and ease of use of the materials in the program or intervention, how well the program or intervention was received by the participants, or an exploration of which groups benefited most from the program or intervention. For example, scientists might interview enrolled subjects following an intervention to better understand their perceptions of the program or intervention, to better understand the utility of the program or intervention, or to understand who is dropping out and why.

A second and likely more frequent use of qualitative methods in community engaged research is with the evaluation of who benefits more (or less) from a community program or intervention. In these evaluations, researchers will sample a subset of participants for interviews to better understand responses to interventions or community programs.

Subsets of participants selected for follow-up interviews might be those who scored high or low on outcome measures. Follow-up interviews for the purpose of gaining a better understanding of study outcomes could be with a convenient sample of participants recruited throughout the study. This option is especially useful when time and resources are limited and when waiting for the conclusion of a study to recruit a select group of high or lower scorers on study outcomes is not feasible.

In the coming chapters, each of the topics summarized here will be discussed in more detail and with specific examples from my own research and that of others. Exemplars chosen are designed to highlight successes, challenges, and lessons learned over the course of my career. It is my hope that you enjoy the work of community-engaged research using qualitative methods as much as I have.

References

Billingsley, A. (1992). *Climbing Jacob's Ladder: The Enduring Legacy of African-American Families*. New York, Simon & Schuster.

Collins, P. H. (1991). *Black Feminist Thought*. New York, Routledge, Chapman and Hall, Inc.

Gamble, V. N. (1993). "A legacy of distrust: African Americans and medical research." *Am J Prev Med* **9**(6 Suppl): 35–38.

Hill, R. B. (1997). *The Strengths of African-American Families: Twenty-Five Years Later*. Baltimore, MD, R & B Publishers.

2 Cultivating and Maintaining Relationships in Community

This chapter focuses on strategies to access underrepresented communities for the purpose of conducting qualitative studies. I specifically focus on strategies used over my 20-year career to develop and maintain collaborative and reciprocal relationships in communities over time. Over the years, I have had the opportunity to collaborate with several communities to conduct qualitative studies. These communities were located in rural and urban areas of the Southern United States including remote rural populations of Southern Appalachia and the coastal areas of North Carolina. While the target populations for my research were individuals who self-identify as African American, and strategies discussed are from that perspective, the information discussed in this chapter is likely applicable to other racial/ethnic populations.

Most Importantly, Do No Harm

As scientists, we are committed to the ethical principal of nonmaleficence (do no harm) in the conduct of research. The principal of doing no harm is particularly relevant when developing collaborative and reciprocal relationships with community and especially relevant during the conduct of qualitative research. A prevailing critique from communities is a sense of feeling abused after granting academic researchers entry to conduct their scientific experiments. Communities report that researchers come into their communities, collect data, and disappear. As a result, communities respond with a greater distrust of researchers and hesitancy to participate in future research studies.

Given the community feedback of a general disrespect among researchers, this entire chapter is devoted to strategies to ensure that science is conducted in a way that shows respect for the community. In this chapter, I describe the strategies I have used to develop and some instances maintain collaborative and reciprocal relationships with communities throughout my career. These strategies include being respectful of the community, keeping your promises to the community, and giving back to the community.

Showing Respect for the Community

During the conduct of qualitative research, scientists may collect data in the private spaces of participant homes and public spaces of faith-based institutions. When entering these spaces, it is critical to be respectful. This respect is inclusive of participant's traditions, values, and history. Respect shown to participants is important even if the qualitative research is conducted in healthcare settings or other public spaces.

DOI: 10.4324/9781003598916-2

Probably the most important display of respect among communities is in the way individuals are addressed during initial interactions. It is important to be familiar with the culture of the community, so stakeholders, community leaders, and potential participants are addressed appropriately. When interacting with community members, I am always careful to know an individual's age, educational degree, and role occupied as leaders in community organizations or in faith-based institutions. The first rule during interactions is that I never address an older person by their first name. Never. Do not ask the individual if it is okay, it is not. In remote rural communities where I was raised, older persons were addressed as Mr. or Mrs., Uncle or Aunt, or Cousin so and so. Older individuals who were close like family members were addressed as Mr. or Miss followed by the first name. Extended older family members were addressed as Aunt or Uncle followed by their first name. Everyone else is addressed as Mr. or Mrs. and their last name. For individuals in faith-based institutions, it is important to understand titles and address individuals appropriately. For example, you may need to address faith-based leaders appropriately as Bishop, Elder, Pastor, or Reverend and Deacon. Some clergy may have earned doctorates in ministry and therefore should be addressed as Dr. followed by their last names. These individuals have worked hard to earn these titles and desire to be appropriately addressed as such.

A second display of respect is in the ways scientists acknowledge that there are formal and informal stakeholders in communities. A formal stakeholder might be the official leader of an organization, and of course, that individual needs to give permission for entry into a community. Formal stakeholders I have had the privilege of working with over the years include Elders of church conferences, Pastors of churches, and Presidents of cancer support groups. These individuals not only are critical to recruitment and enrollment but also an important source of information on the relevance of research questions and study designs.

One long-term research collaboration I have had the pleasure of having was with Sister's Network Triangle, Inc. Early in my research career, I remember talking to friends about a research project that I was interested in pursuing. Fortunately, a friend of a breast cancer survivor invited me to a Sister's Network meeting. I remember attending my first meeting with this group and feeling as though I was an intruder. My goal was to spend time with the group and learn first-hand from them. I wanted to learn more about their social support experiences and whether there were any projects that I might collaborate with them. I remember initially sitting in the back of the room as an observer, but quickly becoming a member of the group—they actually invited me into the group as an Associate member. Over the years, we collaborated on several projects. A relationship that began with me sitting in the back of the room evolved to my being an active member of the group. Although I was never a breast cancer survivor, these women became a huge source of support for me and in my role as a scientist at a predominantly white institution. They were there to help shape my research ideas, to encourage me, and cheer me on as I struggled as an African American scientist on tenure track in a research-intensive environment.

A successful research collaboration may also require relationships with informal stakeholders. Informal stakeholders are individuals who may not be a part of an organization but still have tremendous influence in a community. My experience is that these individuals are longtime residents of a community, and in many ways have given back to community during times of illness and/or financial struggles. Informal stakeholders I have collaborated with had lived in their hometowns the majority of their lives and were longtime members in their churches. These community residents were known for visiting the sick, assisting residents of the community to find work, and sharing their finances with those less fortunate. They were longtime residents of their communities, and their families were also longtime residents. The influence of these informal stakeholders was evident in their own communities but stretched to neighboring counties. One phone call from them to their contacts in neighboring counties was all that was needed for recruitment in those areas. Identifying these informal stakeholders is a time-intensive process, requiring that you get to know the community and spend some time in places they congregate. For my target population, that place was the church. I spent weeks just attending churches, observing social interactions among church congregants to identify these individuals. Just start by introducing yourself, let congregants get to know you, and residents will generally identify and introduce those influential informal stakeholders to you.

Finally, another word about respecting traditions and social norms that may influence your success as a scientist when establishing collaborative community relationships. These traditions and social norms may include how communities celebrate religious traditions, holidays, birthdays, or funerals. Among the communities where I have conducted research, Sundays are generally designated for religious services; Thanksgiving, Christmas, Easter, and the Fourth of July are times of family gatherings and celebrations in African American communities. When recruitment and data collection are scheduled during these dates, I always pause recruiting efforts and data collection to later dates if possible. An interesting recent experience with a mentee was when recruitment numbers decreased during the Christmas Holidays. The mentors and consultants for this project were busy outlining a number of steps the PI should consider while addressing this reduction. I advised the PI to just sit tight until after the holidays. True to my experiences with this population, recruitment picked up after the holidays as I anticipated.

Mealtimes are other considerations. There have been a few times when I scheduled focus groups during the lunch or dinner hour. For these occasions, I always have food, snacks, fruit, and beverages available for participants. However, when traveling to participant's homes, I try to avoid scheduling interviews at high noon or the 5 or 6 pm dinner hour. In addition to not wanting to disrupt mealtimes, I avoid making participants feel obligated to feed me. I did not follow this advice when I first started scheduling interviews. I am not sure if this is still customary, but in previous years in rural communities, it was customary to offer food and drink to visitors. Not wanting to be offensive, I would politely refuse food but always accept something to drink. I frequently tell my students the story of the time I had my young son with me to assist with carrying camera equipment. We arrived at the home of an elderly woman right before the noon lunch hour. When offered food, I politely refused saying that I had a late breakfast. However, the participant looked at my son and said, "Well I know *he's* hungry." She proceeded making my son lunch—a sandwich, drink, and ice cream cup. My son graciously ate what he was given to eat. My son had never eaten a bologna sandwich and did not like ice cream but I was so grateful that for that one time, he ate what he was given.

Keeping Promises

During initial interactions with community, scientists should clearly articulate the purpose of the study in a language familiar to community. Scientists should provide stakeholders and prospective participants with questions they plan to ask, how interviews will be conducted, and most importantly, who will see their information and how that information will be used. I have generally included a little about myself and the reasons for my interests in their stories. For example, in one study designed to better understand the uses of religious songs during life-threatening illness, I informed potential participants that I was a nursing professor at the University of North Carolina at Chapel Hill, born and raised in the Western part of North Carolina, graduated from local universities, and attended a local church. So, although I was affiliated with a predominantly white university, I had affiliations with organizations in the community. My interest in the topic was clearly articulated as wanting to document the positive uses of religious songs in response to life-threatening illness of oneself, close family member, or the death of a family member. This explanation was adequate for stakeholders of communities in well-educated urban populations, but I needed an expanded strategy for stakeholders of more remote, rural communities who had never participated in a research study. For stakeholders of these remote and rural communities, I would go through the process of enrollment and data collection, or simply allow the stakeholder to sit in on the interview. This process was beneficial in showing stakeholders that I would only ask questions as promised.

Promises related to time and incentives should also be respected. Show up as promised, stay only as long as promised, and distribute incentives as promised. Showing up as promised is simply being on time to appointments. If you need to cancel, arrange for someone else to go in your place. They may have rearranged their day to accommodate your visit, and they should be your priority. When traveling in remote rural areas on roads I am not familiar with, or even when I find myself stuck in traffic or behind a slow-driving car on a two-lane country road, I pull over and phone ahead to let the participant know that I will be late and why. I have been late to more than one appointment because I made a wrong turn (Google Maps was confused). When I arrived, the participant was sitting outside in a lawn chair waiting for me. Oftentimes, for older participants in the country, you may be their only visitor for the day, and they will be waiting for you to show up.

Do not exceed the time you told them it would take to conduct the interview. If the interview is taking longer than expected, remember you are changing your contract with them. Any changes to what you told them about the interview need to be renegotiated. It is always good practice to get their permission to stay longer than planned. While it may appear that participants are enjoying the interview and just now opening up about their experiences, they will remember that you stayed longer than you said potentially keeping them from other activities they had planned for the day. Better to pause and get permission to stay longer, or even better, arrange for a second follow-up interview. I have done these follow-up interviews by phone, which has worked well.

A final word about the distribution of incentives in communities. If possible, incentives paid in cash (not checks) are best. I was once recruiting a very low-income and older urban population, and the preferred option for cash incentives at my institution was to distribute checks. Among this low-income population, cashing a check would have likely entailed a trip to a local convenience store or check-cashing store that charges fees for their services. I pushed back and was granted permission to distribute cash. The distribution of cash required extra security measures and record keeping but better for the burden of incentives to be placed among the researcher's team than the participants. The distribution of incentives in the form of gift cards is less burdensome than cash. However, for gift cards to be usable, the researcher needs some knowledge of the physical environment of the community. For example, I was once distributing Walmart cards to an older population which was fine for a younger population or others without physical limitations. Older participants in remote rural areas were not able to drive 10–14 miles to Walmart. Because of this, they preferred a gift card to the grocery chain in their neighborhoods, stores that were more accessible. Lastly, I have always distributed any incentive prior to the start of the interview. That is, when asking participants to sign the consent form, I go ahead and have them sign for the incentive so that the remainder of our time is focused on the interview. My rationale for distributing incentives prior to the interview is that they are not distracted during the interview, wondering whether you are really going to give them what you have promised. In my twenty years as a scientist, I have never distributed an incentive and not completed an interview.

Although not a promise to community, I felt it was important to disseminate the findings back to the community. The purpose of disseminating back to the community was to let them see how their stories were used and to also give them access to their stories for their own use. For example, I have given community members copies of papers published in academic journals that they would otherwise not have access to. I also agreed to and presented findings to community-sponsored educational programs and health fairs. However, I regret not being able to disseminate the findings back to communities in remote rural areas. My long-term goal is to write a book about these stories that can be available to the lay public, stories that will reach these communities.

Giving Back to the Community

Contributing your knowledge and skills. Researchers generally think of reciprocity in community-engaged research as paying incentives or paying advisory board members for their time and efforts in ensuring the success of the project. Monetary incentives given to participants are nice and additional stipends to churches even nicer, but the best contribution is when a scientist contributes their knowledge, skills, or financial resources to benefit the community after the project has ended. Very few community-engaged researchers commit to long-term collaborative relationships or return to the community to truly give back in this way.

Contributing your knowledge and skillset. Scientists in the academy generally hold advanced degrees in the health sciences such as medicine, nursing, and public health. Nurses and physicians may also be certified practitioners in their respective fields. Important to note as well is that many senior scientists (particularly those of color) may be the first in the families to attend college and one of the less than 2% to achieve the rank of professor in their discipline. When engaging with communities using qualitative methods, I always remember the folk that encouraged and supported me along this journey and the obligation that I have to give back to individuals like those who made my success in the academy possible. As an academic partner with a program of research focused on the social support experiences of cancer survivors, I participated in community outreach activities of a breast cancer support group through my participation in sponsored symposiums and through financial contributions to fundraisers. For example, I was invited to speak at the "Spirituality and Cancer" Sisters Network 10th Annual Surviving & Thriving Symposium." A second instance of using my knowledge to give back to the community was through a research class offered to a small group of Sister's Network members. In this class, I educated these women about research terminology and the process of a research study so that they would be more informed and able to advocate for their organization when approached by scientists wanting to engage them in research.

As healthcare practitioners, we might consider contributing our skills to community events that promote cancer screenings, mental health awareness, substance abuse educational sessions, or even smoking cessation events.

Contributing financial resources. As scientists, we may have access to financial resources that we can share with the community. For example, I have been able to use my discretionary funds to purchase tickets for the Sister's Network Annual Tea Event and gift these tickets to enable other members so they can attend as well. Over the years, I have also contributed Walmart cards to the Health and Wellness committee of Sister's Network Triangle. The Health and Wellness committee used these gift cards to relieve some of the financial burden on members in treatment, assisting them to buy gas, medications, or food. I wish I would have done more but I did what I could at the time. Although I live elsewhere, during the COVID pandemic, I contributed financially to the small churches in rural areas who were threatened with the possibility of having to close their doors permanently when offerings and tithes were decreased.

Conclusion

Community-engaged research combined with qualitative methods is extremely time-intensive. Building relationships is time-consuming but extremely rewarding. The strategies put forth in this chapter are those that I have learned over the years and will hopefully make your journey easier.

3 Research Questions Appropriate for SDOH and Qualitative Methods

This chapter is an overview of research questions that guide the use of qualitative methods. I also include a rationale (the problem) associated with the exemplar research questions. Specifically, I describe research questions that potentially guide the study designs listed below:

- Exploratory studies
  - Grounded theory
  - Phenomenology
  - Ethnography
  - Narrative analysis
  - Qualitative descriptive
- Pilot or preliminary studies
  - Development/adapting instruments for underrepresented populations in communities
  - Development of interventions for underrepresented populations in communities
  - Evaluation of intervention processes

In the majority of research projects that I have led, I have used qualitative methods prior to, during, or following measurement and intervention studies. In this chapter, I will discuss my experiences using qualitative methods with these SDOH-focused research projects and offer insights into appropriate research questions for the designs used in these studies. In later chapters, I will describe ways in which I have used theory, sampling strategies, data collection, and data analysis for the research questions using exemplar projects described in this chapter. The exemplar research projects described in this chapter are those for which I was the Principal Investigator or mentor. This approach to the selection of exemplar cases permits a more in-depth description of the topics related to SDOH and other related topics discussed throughout this book.

Exploratory Studies

As mentioned in Chapter 2, my segue into the conduct of qualitative research was to better understand the social support experiences of older African American cancer patients. From the qualitative approaches of grounded theory, phenomenology, ethnography, narrative analysis, and descriptive qualitative approaches, I selected the grounded theory approach as the most appropriate to answer the research question for this particular study. In this first section on exploratory studies, I briefly review a selection of qualitative

DOI: 10.4324/9781003598916-3

approaches to explain my rationale for the utilization of one approach over the other. I begin the discussion with the qualitative approach of grounded theory.

Grounded theory was the method selected to guide the study titled "Theorizing social support among African American Cancer Survivors (Hamilton, 2001)."Grounded theory as an approach to qualitative research originated in the discipline of sociology. This approach seeks to guide studies that have the purpose of generating a tentative theory or typology of categories related to social interactions. It is an exploration of how individuals make sense of a process (Strauss & Corbin, 1990). Grounded theory was appropriate given the purpose of this study to understand supportive interactions and to develop a culturally relevant theory of social support for African Americans. Grounded theory was used to guide this in-depth exploration of social support as a social construct. It was further used to discover the events, actions, and behaviors that expanded what was known of this phenomenon. Specifically, this approach permitted an in-depth exploration of social support experiences among older African American cancer patients as interview questions were centered around events leading up to the use of a type of social support (the antecedent influence), the social support experience (major category), and the outcome from the social support experience (the consequence). This in-depth exploration, along with the systematic process of simultaneous data collection and analysis, guided the formulation of relationships among newly discovered concepts into an explanatory framework for the development of a theory of social support.

Example 1. Theorizing Social Support Among African American Cancer Survivors

Theorizing social support among African American cancer survivors was my dissertation research and the foundation for research conducted throughout my career (Hamilton, 2001). Moreover, during this project, I received mentoring on how to conduct qualitative research using rigorous methodologies.

The purpose of this study was to explore the meaning of social support from the perspective of African Americans with cancer. Using a grounded theory approach, I explored conceptualizations and uses of social support from the perspective of African American men treated for prostate cancer and African American women treated for breast cancer. The immediate goal of this study was to develop an understanding of the meaning of social support from the perspective of African Americans diagnosed with cancer.

The research questions addressed in this study were (1) How do African Americans with cancer understand social support; for example, what language do they use, and how do they conceive it? (2) What are the social support resources available to and used by African Americans with cancer? (3) What are those factors that influence the use of social support resources by African Americans with cancer? (4) What are the outcomes or consequences of the use of social support among this population? and (5) How do African Americans use social support to cope with their cancer experience that extends through treatment and the aftermath of treatment?

The problem was derived from the increased burden of cancer among African Americans. African Americans continue to have the highest overall incidence of cancer than any other racial or ethnic group in the United States (Saka et al., 2025). Although the American Cancer Society has reported a decline in cancer deaths for African Americans, the cancer mortality rates for African Americans are still 33% higher than those for Caucasians and twice as high as those for all other U.S. minority populations (Saka et al., 2025). When the diagnosis is breast cancer, African American women have the highest mortality rates of all racial and ethnic groups. African American men are more than twice as likely to die of prostate cancer as any other racial or ethnic group (Saka et al., 2025). Additionally, African Americans with cancer have shorter survival rates than whites at all stages (Saka et al., 2025). To compound this disproportionate cancer burden, African Americans are more likely to enter treatment with more advanced diagnostic staging (Saka et al., 2025). Entering treatment when diagnosed with later staging can translate into a poorer diagnosis with increased morbidity and psychological distress that is associated with more advanced cancer treatments. Although African Americans have the worst morbidity and mortality rates of any group with cancer, few social support studies have included African Americans diagnosed with cancer.

Phenomenology—A second qualitative approach I could have used to understand the experience of social support among African American cancer survivors could have been through phenomenology. Using phenomenology, an appropriate research question would be "What is the lived experience of social support for older African Americans when receiving chemotherapy for treatment of cancer?" I would be specifically exploring feelings associated with the receipt of social support for African Americans when receiving chemotherapy as a treatment for cancer.

Phenomenology is an approach to qualitative research with the purpose of a social phenomenon (subjective point of view) as it is immediately experienced (Drake et al., 2025). Proponents of this tradition argued for a method that captured an experiential world focused on a subjective real-life experience (Drake et al., 2025). It is also important to note that with this tradition, the phenomenon of interest must be a conscious experience as it is encountered. In contrast to the grounded theory approach that asks questions related to who did what? When? Where? How many? Under what conditions? research questions using the phenomenological tradition ask the question related to what it is, what it says, and how it speaks. Further, in contrast to grounded theory, phenomenology is not used to identify a taxonomy of concepts or an abstract tentative theory. Given the interest in the social support experiences of older African American cancer patients, phenomenology would have been useful to guide an exploration of how social support was experienced during a specific event. It would provide a better understanding in real-time of the emotions such as fears, anxieties, or even depressed moods that shaped the social interactions of giving and receiving social support. An example purpose statement might be to explore how older African American cancer patients experience social interactions among family members and the social support derived from these interactions during a cancer treatment.

Ethnography—A third qualitative approach I could have used to understand the experience of social support among African American cancer survivors could have been through an ethnographic tradition. Using ethnography, an appropriate research question would be "How is social support experienced among African Americans as congregants of faith-based institutions in a rural isolated community in the Southern Appalachian region? or "How do church congregants respond to the news of a cancer diagnosis of older African American clergy?"

Ethnography is an approach to qualitative research that originated in the discipline of anthropology and seeks to guide studies that have the purpose of understanding cultures, individual ways of living, believing, and adapting. This tradition further emphasizes and builds on perspectives of participants in a given setting. Ethnography is further described as a tradition that seeks to understand how individuals make meaning of their lives, one that is highly variable and specific to a local community (LeCompte & Schensul, 1999). In

comparison to grounded theory, ethnography can be used to guide the building of a local theory or adapting a theory for use among different populations. On the other hand, in contrast to phenomenology, studies using an ethnographic tradition focus on the understanding of the culture of a community and its members in a specific setting (LeCompte & Schensul, 1999). Again, using the problem that little is known of the social support experiences of older African American cancer patients, and with interest in the social support networks among this population, ethnography would be an appropriate qualitative method. Ethnography is appropriate to understand the culture of supportive (or not) interactions among congregants and clergy in a natural setting (the church). In comparison to grounded theory and phenomenology, where the perspective of an individual is explored, ethnography would permit for the collective of experiences—the congregants as givers of support and the clergy as recipients of support, or a congregant as receiver and clergy as giver. It is important, however, to explore perspectives of when support is given (or not) and when support is received (or not) as well as the context for the giving and receiving of support, who is involved, what are the beliefs around giving and receiving support, and what are the types of social support given during interactions among congregants and clergy. As you can tell, an ethnographic study can be quite time-intensive and include a combination of observation and interviews.

Narrative methods—A fourth qualitative approach I could have used to understand the experience of social support among African American cancer survivors is through narrative analysis approach. Example research questions might be "How is the story told?," "What contributed to my cancer diagnosis?" or maybe "How did this cancer diagnosis change me?"

Narrative analysis is a qualitative approach that is frequently used in anthropology, history, and literature and seeks to understand how individuals and communities attribute causality for their experiences (Riessman, 2008). The tradition of narrative methods is an approach to data analysis that seeks to explore personal meanings from a collection of personal stories; how individuals make sense of their experience; or how stories have shaped individual identities in response to some event or experience (Riessman, 2008). Narrative methods are well-suited for SDOH research using qualitative methods since this tradition assumes that stories have a social, cultural, and historical context that shapes the ways in which individuals make sense of their lives. Similar to the other traditions, this tradition is useful to guide research using qualitative methods in explorations of SDOH in communities to understand individual experiences (Riessman, 2008; Schensul et al., 1999)). However, the benefit of narrative analysis is in the approach to analyzing collected stories for the way individuals construct the stories, and identities, around their experiences.

In the interviews conducted to better understand the social support experiences of older African American cancer patients, a narrative analysis could be used to guide a further exploration of how their experience with cancer and social support shaped their identities. Narrative analysis might also be used to guide an exploration of the stories to better understand the historical influences on the types of social support given and received during a cancer diagnosis or an understanding of the ways their experiences with other cancer survivors shaped their willingness to ask for or receive social support when diagnosed with cancer. Narrative analysis has been useful in my own program of research when developing intervention vignettes to capture individual experiences with cancer survivorship in a story. For example, how the story evolved from the beginning, middle, and end with characters and a plot that resulted in a story to persuade or engage others to change some behavior.

Qualitative descriptive—This approach would have been useful to guide research to understand the process of exchanging social support among networks of family and friends of older African American cancer patients.

Perhaps the most frequently used qualitative research tradition is qualitative description (Sandelowski, 2000, 2010). This tradition is useful when seeking to solely describe a phenomenon. Qualitative descriptive tradition may lack interpretative depth and may not be linked to any of the other traditions. In comparison to grounded theory, phenomenology, ethnography, or narrative methods, the qualitative descriptive approach is viewed as a less rigorous approach, less interpretative, and lacking a conceptual or highly abstract rendering. Given the more concrete and factual nature of the qualitative descriptive approach, research using this tradition may be less time-intensive and therefore more desirable for preliminary studies or studies using mixed methods.

In my own research, I have used a qualitative descriptive design to guide research that seeks to understand the social determinants of the outcome variable psychological distress. A review of the literature on this topic suggests African Americans continue to experience the highest overall cancer mortality rates, more advanced-staged cancers (American Cancer Society, 2025), and higher levels of psychological distress from cancer than non-Hispanic Whites (Alcala, 2014). High levels of psychological distress among African Americans have been linked to unmet needs for support and information from healthcare providers (Sklenarova et al., 2015). Additionally, the root cause of psychological distress among this population has been attributed to overwhelming anxieties and concerns that cancer will lead to suffering, death, and isolation for their family member diagnosed with cancer (Hamilton et al., 2015; Rositch et al., 2019; Schoenfeld & Francis, 2016). Despite high levels of psychological distress, African American patients and family members are not likely to seek mental health services (Traeger et al., 2014) or to participate in support groups (Somayaji & Cloyes, 2015). African American cancer patients and family members report being receptive to interventions that incorporate cognitive and culturally-based strategies (Hamilton et al., 2015), yet these interventions lack conceptual clarity and are rarely tailored for diverse populations (Balboni et al., 2017).

Example 2. Social Support and Psychological Distress among Older African American Cancer Survivors

The purpose of this study was to explore the perceptions of psychological distress among older adult African American cancer survivors. The specific goals of this project were to increase my understanding of experienced psychological distress among cancer survivors engaged in giving and receiving social support from their social networks of family and friends.

The research question for this project was "What are perceptions of psychological distress among African American cancer survivors engaged in social support interactions among family and friends?" My interest in this topic was derived from the low scores reported among African American cancer survivors on the Hospital Anxiety and Depression Scale (HADS) during one of my quantitative projects. I was particularly interested in conducting this qualitative study for two reasons. First, the prevailing research suggests that in comparison with other racial/ethnic groups, African American cancer patients are more likely to experience high levels of psychological distress. Secondly, the HADS is a well-known and frequently used measure of psychological distress. It is the gold standard from which the majority of our knowledge on distress is derived.

Preliminary or Pilot Studies

In addition to using qualitative methods to explore perceptions of understudied topics or to enhance one's understanding of a problem in an understudied population, this research design is useful when developing or adapting measures, and or developing or adapting interventions.

Qualitative Methods to Support the Development of Measures and Interventions

In measurement studies, qualitative methods are useful in the development of new measures to capture a previously unmeasured concept or to adapt existing measures for use in a different target population. When the end goal of a research project is an intervention, qualitative methods are useful to identify appropriate components of the intervention, the feasibility of the intervention, and to understand processes of the intervention or an understanding of outcomes.

In the next two sections, I describe the ways in which I used qualitative methods to develop a measure of social support and a storytelling intervention. The qualitative research supported an NIH R01-funded study for a new measure of social support and an NIH-funded R03 study for the development of a storytelling intervention to alleviate psychological distress among African American cancer survivors.

Development of the Ways of Helping Questionnaire: A Measure of Preferred Coping Strategies for Older African American Cancer Survivors

As previously discussed in this chapter, a grounded theory study designed to better understand the social support experiences of an older African American cancer population led to a new conceptualization of social support and subsequently the development of a new measure of social support (Hamilton et al., 2009). The new measure, the Ways of Helping Questionnaire, was guided by a qualitative method using grounded theory to generate a typology of social support that was the foundation of this new measure. The Ways of Helping Questionnaire addressed several weaknesses of existing social support measures but also captured the strengths of social support among African American cancer survivors.

First, existing measures lacked a focus on social support from God as a Deity. The support available from a perceived immortal and all-powerful source is perceived to send help not available through mortal beings (Hamilton et al., 2007). For example, God is perceived to provide the social support of comfort, strengthening familial relationships, a refuge for confiding and consulting with worries and treatment-related decisions, and a trusted resource for alleviating worries (Hamilton et al., 2007).

Secondly, existing measures failed to capture the social support available through an elaborate system of mutual aid among family, friends, and fellow church congregants. This system of mutual aid provides for the collective pooling of resources to assist community members in times of need. Lastly, items in existing social support measures were generally written in a language or vernacular not used or unfamiliar to the culture of older African Americans (Hamilton et al., 2009). Therefore, the findings of this qualitative study suggested the necessity to develop a new measure of social support that included types of social support missing in existing measures. We discuss in more detail in later chapters the conceptualizations, sampling strategy, data collection, and data analysis used in this qualitative study.

Qualitative research methods are quite useful in adapting instruments to be more culturally relevant for underserved populations. Adapting of measures is less costly and less time-consuming than the process of developing a new measure. Further, adapting a measure is much more practical and feasible when researchers need to quickly move to an experimental design or intervention study. Considerations for adapting an existing measure might be for a revision in the language being used, the need to modify content, or to rewrite items for a more appropriate reading level.

For example, I once modified a 15-item Mutuality scale designed for use with family caregivers and their frail or ill older relatives (Archbold et al., 1990). While the original scale was written to capture content focused on caregiving, I found that the items could easily be reworded to capture the relationship well-being between participants and their family and friends, and therefore appropriate for a quantitative study to examine the construct validity of the Ways of Helping Questionnaire. Items in the original scale were worded to capture the perspective and value of a familial vs individualistic lens. An original item "How often do you feel physically close to him or her" was reworded "How close do you feel to your family since your illness." A second item, "How much do you confide in him or her?" was reworded "How much do you talk to family about your illness?" captured the familial perspective but used language (talk vs confide) generally used in daily conversation among older African Americans. And, finally, an original item "How much love do you feel for him or her" reworded "How much do you feel your family is there for you" captured the frequent expression among cancer survivors. The emotion of feeling supported when family "was there for me" was captured in research.

Messages of Hope Intervention Development

As I was completing the Ways of Helping Measurement Study, I realized that another pressing research was the need for an understanding of the experiences of those African American cancer survivors who were lacking the support from a network of close family, extended family, friends, and fellow church congregants. The literature has suggested that there is a general lack of social support for this African American population and while my earlier research suggested that social support was forthcoming for many, I needed to understand the context for when support was absent. Qualitative methods using grounded theory techniques used again to guide a research project to understand the perceived social support needs among older adult African American cancer survivors.

Example 3. Messages of Hope: Helping Family Members to Overcome Fears and Fatalistic Attitudes toward Cancer

This study was conducted to explore the perspectives of fears and fatalistic attitudes toward a cancer diagnosis among family members of African American patients and to identify strategies used among this population to overcome those fears (Hamilton et al., 2017). The research question guiding this qualitative study was "What are the perceived fears and fatalistic attitudes among family members of cancer patients during treatment?" A second research question guiding this qualitative study was "What are the strategies used among family members of African American cancer patients to overcome fears and fatalistic attitudes toward cancer?"

The problem for this study was derived from evidence that intergenerational stories that have generated fears and fatalistic attitudes toward cancer have been extremely detrimental to African American health and disparities, significantly decreasing participation in early detection programs, the access of timely and optimal cancer care and ultimately contributing to high cancer mortality rates (Hamilton et al., 2017). Moreover, when cancer patients are fearful and assume they will be socially isolated within their communities, they may not disclose a cancer diagnosis which limits the social support available to them (Hamilton et al., 2017). Older African Americans have identified the root causes of fears and fatalistic attitudes toward cancer within their communities as the result of (1) past experiences of seeing or hearing about individuals who died a painful and disfiguring death; (2) a culture whereby cancer was not openly discussed; and (3) limited exposure to African American cancer survivors who successfully maintained roles at home and work (Hamilton et al., 2017). Interventions specifically designed to address fears and fatalistic attitudes toward cancer are limited to culturally targeted educational booklets to enhance cancer awareness and participation in early detection programs. These studies do not address the distress and fears experienced among individuals with a confirmed cancer diagnosis. In addition, interventions delivered solely through printed materials may not be usable among older African Americans with limited opportunities for a formal education and low reading levels.

The findings from this qualitative research contributed to the evidence needed to reduce cancer disparities through the development of an innovative intervention using an interactive DVD of messages of hope using religious songs and scripture. This interactive DVD consists of testimonials (positive cancer survivorship stories) from older African American cancer survivors who shared their survivorship stories to enable other patients in being less fearful, comforted, and ultimately persevere through prescribed cancer treatments (16–18). African Americans have a strong culture of being in service to others during adversity, and it is therefore imperative that we integrate this important cultural aspect into interventions targeting this population, with the ultimate goal of reducing health disparities.

Qualitative Research to Evaluate Intervention Processes and Outcomes

In this final section on research questions appropriate to qualitative methods, I present my experience with two projects to explore participants' perceptions of the intervention's delivery and context within which desired outcomes were achieved or not. Specifically, the focus in this section is on explorations of participant perceptions of the processes and outcomes of a culturally relevant cancer survivorship storytelling intervention. This exemplar study permits an in-depth description of the ways in which qualitative methods can provide the data that enables the research team to understand the context within which the intervention was acceptable and feasible for the intended target population. Secondly, this qualitative exploration provided insights into the context of which participants benefit (or not) from the intervention.

The exemplar study is the *Faith-based African American Cancer Survivorship Stories Intervention*. This intervention was developed to provide positive stories of cancer survivorship to African American cancer patients and their family members. We anticipated that the Faith-based African American Cancer Survivorship Stories would be emotionally engaging for the study participants since storytelling is an important aspect of the cultural history of this population. Although storytelling as a strategy to communicate hope during adversity is a strategy familiar to this population, particularly when faced with a new and very distressful situation such as cancer. We anticipated that through the process of transportation, participants would relate these stories to their own experiences and *engage in discussions* on ways in which a positive survivorship story might be used to decrease psychological distress.

The research questions guiding the qualitative aim of this project were "Will a Faith-based African American Cancer Survivorship Stories Intervention be feasible and acceptable?" and "How do participants describe the impact of this intervention on their psychological distress"?

Conclusion

In this chapter, I discuss the research question driving research projects focused on SDOH using qualitative research methods. The use of conceptualizations, theory, sampling strategies, data collection, and data analysis of these exemplar qualitative studies will be described in detail in future chapters.

References

Alcala, H. E. (2014). "Differential mental health impact of cancer across racial/ethnic groups: Findings from a population-based study in California." *BMC Public Health* **14**: 930.

American Cancer Society. (2025). *Cancer Statistics for African American and Black People, 2025*. Atlanta, American Cancer Society.

Archbold, P. G., B. J. Stewart, M. R. Greenlick and T. Harvath. (1990). "Mutuality and preparedness as predictors of caregiver role strain." *Res Nurs Health* **13**(6): 375–384.

Balboni, T. A., G. Fitchett, G. F. Handzo, K. S. Johnson, H. G. Koenig, K. I. Pargament, C. M. Puchalski, S. Sinclair, E. J. Taylor and K. E. Steinhauser. (2017). "State of the science of spirituality and palliative care research part II: Screening, assessment, and interventions." *J Pain Symptom Manag* **54**(3): 441–453.

Drake, E. K., L. E. Weeks, D. Taylor, I. Ricci, J. Curran and M. van Manen (2025). "Engaging in palliative care conversations with healthcare providers: A phenomenological young adult cancer study." *Qual Health Res*. 28:10497323251325471. Epub ahead of print. doi: 10.1177/10497323251325471

Hamilton, J. (2001). *Theorizing Social Support among African Americans with Cancer*. Doctoral Dissertation. Chapel Hill, North Carolina, University of North Carolina.

Hamilton, J., B. Powe, A. Pollard, K. Lee and A. Felton. (2007). "Spirituality among African American cancer survivors." *Cancer Nurs* **30**(3): 309–316.

Hamilton, J. B., B. J. Stewart, J. L. Crandell and M. R. Lynn. (2009). "Development of the ways of helping questionnaire: A measure of preferred coping strategies for older African American cancer survivors." *Res Nurs Health* **32**(3): 243–259.

Hamilton, J. B., V. C. Worthy, A. D. Moore, N. C. Best, J. M. Stewart and M. K. Song. (2017). "Messages of hope: Helping family members to overcome fears and fatalistic attitudes toward cancer." *J Cancer Educ* **32**(1): 190–197.

LeCompte, M. D. and J. J. Schensul. (1999). *Designing and Conducting Ethnographic Research*. Walnut Creek, CA, AltaMira Press.

Riessman, C. K. (2008). *Narrative Methods for the Human Science*. Los Angeles, CA, Sage Publishing.

Rositch, A. F., R. Atnafou, M. Krakow and G. D'Souza (2019). "A community-based qualitative assessment of knowledge, barriers, and promoters of communicating about family cancer history among African-Americans." *Health Commun* **34**(10): 1192–1201. doi: 10.1080/10410236.2018.1471335

Saka, A. H., A. N. Giaquinto, L. E. McCullough, K. Y. Tossas, J. Star, A. Jemal and R. L. Siegel. (2025). "Cancer statistics for African American and Black people, 2025." *CA: Cancer J Clini* **75**(2): 111–140.

Sandelowski, M. (2000). "Whatever happened to qualitative description?" *Res Nurs Health* **23**: 334–340.

Sandelowski, M. (2010). "What's in a name? Qualitative description revisited." *Res Nurs Health* **33**(1): 77–84.

Schensul, S. L., J. J. Schensul and M. D. LeCompte (1999). Essential ethnographic methods: Observation, interviews, and questionnaires. Walnut Creek, CA, Altamira Press. A Division of Sage Publications Inc.

Schoenfeld, E. R. and L. E. Francis. (2016). "Word on the street: Engaging local leaders in a dialogue about prostate cancer among African Americans." *Am J Mens Health* **10**(5): 377–388.

Sklenarova, H., A. Krumpelmann, M. W. Haun, H. C. Friederich, J. Huber, M. Thomas, E. C. Winkler, W. Herzog and M. Hartmann. (2015). "When do we need to care about the caregiver? Supportive care needs, anxiety, and depression among informal caregivers of patients with cancer and cancer survivors." *Cancer* **121**(9): 1513–1519.

Somayaji, D. and K. G. Cloyes. (2015). "Cancer fear and fatalism: How African American participants construct the role of research subject in relation to clinical cancer research." *Cancer Nurs* **38**(2): 133–144.

Strauss, A. and J. Corbin. (1990). *Basics of Qualitative Research: Grounded Theory Procedures and Techniques*. Newbury Park, CA, Sage.

Traeger, L., S. Cannon, N. L. Keating, W. F. Pirl, C. Lathan, M. Y. Martin, Y. He and E. R. Park. (2014). "Race by sex differences in depression symptoms and psychosocial service use among non-Hispanic black and white patients with lung cancer." *J Clin Oncol* **32**(2): 107–113.

4 The Use of Conceptualizations and Theories with Qualitative Methods

Theory is the lens through which we understand or gain insight into a phenomenon. Scholars generally agree that a clearly articulated conceptualization, conceptual framework, or theory is critical to well-designed and rigorously executed quantitative and qualitative research projects. Although these research tools are critical to both quantitative and qualitative methods, there are differences in the ways they are used. Quantitative researchers generally use conceptual frameworks and theories to explain hypotheses, predict outcomes, guide data collection methods, and interpret findings. On the other hand, qualitative researchers use conceptualizations and/or theories as a theoretical lens by which they understand a phenomenon, selecting the appropriate qualitative approach, the sampling strategies, interview questions, analyze data, and interpret and present findings.

Qualitative researchers may begin a study opting to allow a theory or framework to emerge during the study. Scholars of qualitative methodology have argued that a theoretical framework is not necessary at the outset of a qualitative study; however, I would argue that theory drives all research. And, even when theory is not explicitly stated, it is critical to have a clearly articulated conceptualization of the phenomenon of interest. A frequent practice among qualitative researchers, particularly those beginning this area of inquiry, is the insertion of a theoretical or conceptual framework in a diagram with all the blocks and arrows that illustrate the direction or associations among variables. This is confusing at best and even an inappropriate use of theory. In this chapter, I describe the ways in which I have used theory as a lens or way of thinking about a phenomenon in my program of research. To achieve this goal, I will use two exemplar studies. In this first example, I describe in detail the ways in which a theory emerged from the findings.

Example 1. Theorizing Social Support Among African American Cancer Patients

As mentioned in Chapter 3, the purpose of the qualitative project "Theorizing Social Support among African American Cancer Patients" was to explore the meaning of social support from the perspective of this population. Using a grounded theory approach, I explored conceptualizations of social support from the perspective of African American men treated for prostate cancer and African American women treated for breast cancer. The immediate goal of this study was to develop an understanding of the meaning of social support from the perspective of African Americans diagnosed with cancer. Although I did not use an explicitly stated theory to guide this study, I was sensitized to conceptualizations of social support through existing literature. Which brings to mind another question. How is literature used in a qualitative study? As you will read, I review literature prior to conducting a study, during a study, and again during the interpretation of findings and

DOI: 10.4324/9781003598916-4

when writing the discussion section of a manuscript. The literature reviewed changes during the course of a study, and I have frequently found it necessary to read outside of the health sciences to understand the role of culture in the lived experiences of African Americans.

A review of the literature demonstrated that social support was informative in the ways social support research has focused on two areas: (1) the types and amounts of social support exchanged and (2) the social networks through which social support is exchanged. According to the literature reviewed in the health sciences and sociology, social support is a resource provided by social networks, that is primarily conceptualized into three categories: (1) emotional support; (2) instrumental support; and (3) informational support (Helgeson & Cohen, 1996; House & Kahn, 1985; Tilden, 1985). The most frequently studied emotional support is the open expression of love and/or liking and active listening to worries and concerns. Another conceptualization of emotional support, sometimes referred to as appraisal support, involves being valued, esteemed, and provided feedback about one's self-worth. Instrumental support, the second category of social support, is also referred to as tangible support, the act of providing material aid or assistance with finances, household tasks, goods, and services. Informational support is a third category of social support that entails or involves assistance in obtaining information or advice about some problem or illness.

Prevailing conceptualizations of social support (emotional, instrumental, informational) generated from research conducted among predominantly white middle-class populations were problematic when applied to African Americans for several reasons. Primarily, when African Americans have been included in this body of research, scholars have made comparisons to white populations and concluded that African Americans are lacking in social support. When comparisons have been made using prevailing conceptualizations of social support, one conclusion has been that African Americans have lower amounts of emotional support. Specifically, this conclusion comes from the conceptualization of emotional support as the open expression of love and confiding in family and friends about health-related problems. However, in evidence generated from historical and cultural studies, African Americans themselves report having emotional support. According to this literature, emotional support is in the form of companionship, encouragement, kind words and gestures (Chatters et al., 1994; Jayakody et al., 1993); not necessarily open expressions of love. Additionally, the depiction of African Americans lacking emotional support originated from research findings that revealed lower amounts of confiding support in this population. African Americans, however, have been less likely to discuss certain types of problems with members of their social networks (Chatters et al., 1994; Degazon, 1994; Ellison, 1995). Scholars have generally accepted these findings as truths and not engaged in the research to determine the strengths of this population. In other words, scholars have focused on what is not there, rather than what is there.

Once I expanded my reading of the literature in the anthropology and historical literature, I became more aware of the strengths of African American populations. This expanding review of the literature captured the voices of African Americans, their experiences with social support, and the many documented instances of a mutual aid system that actively responds to the problems African Americans through sharing resources in times of need. The existence of this mutual aid system suggests that the social networks that provide social support to African Americans extend beyond the immediate nuclear family and known networks of family and friends. Largely ignored in health and illness literature, this mutual aid system has functioned successfully for generations in the survival of African American families. It is important now to know how it functions as a source of social support when the adverse situation is a life-threatening illness.

In the beginning of this project, I was sensitized to a body of scientific literature where social support researchers have focused on weaknesses and deficiencies among African American cancer patients in their social networks and social support. During reading from the disciplines of history and anthropology, I was also aware that social support research has primarily ignored the cultural relevance of this construct among African American cancer populations but largely ignored a history of mutual aid and assistance that has served as a buffer against institutional slavery, oppression, and other atrocities this population has endured. A culturally applicable understanding of social support among African Americans is needed in order to properly appraise the utility of this concept with this ethnic minority population. Since social support as measured in the majority population has been found to be an important coping strategy, it is crucial to know if this concept is equally important for African Americans with cancer.

Moving Forward with a Culturally Relevant Conceptualization of Social Support

The findings from this qualitative research project using a grounded theory approach resulted in additional categories of social support (I discuss the analysis of the data in Chapter 8). See Table 4.1.

Table 4.1 Definitions of Types of Social Support

Category	*Subcategory*	*Definition*
Emotional support	Presence of others	A communication of verbal and nonverbal behaviors from network members that they are available and willing to help in whatever way needed; a form of companionship.
	Encouraging words	A verbal communication from network members the cancer patient perceives as positive, uplifting, motivating; to reassure or to encourage positive self-evaluation.
	Distracting activities	Diversionary activities provided by network members; Behaviors from network members to divert the cancer patient's mind from the cancer experience and related problems or concerns.
	Protecting/monitoring	Actions or behaviors done to guard, shield someone against something. To protect from further harm.
Instrumental support	Offers of prayers	Any communication from social network members that they are praying for the cancer patient.
	Assistance to maintain social roles	Assistance from network members to help the cancer patient maintain social roles in their workplace, churches, or families/homes.
	Assistance to continue religious practices	Support from network members to assist the cancer patient in continuing religious practices—Holy Communion, tithing, conducting religious services outside of the church.
	Assistance to continue living in the home.	Having network members move in permanently or temporarily to allow the cancer patient to continue living at home.
Informational support		Similar to existing definitions of informational support. Includes help to understand information, and advice, validating information received. Also includes assistance to select physician or treatment facility.

Table 4.2 Comparison of Conceptualizations of Social Support

Existing conceptualization	*Culturally relevant conceptualization*
Emotional Support	*Emotional Support*
• Expressions of liking, love, listening to worries and concerns • Confiding in family and friends about problems	• Presence of others • Encouraging words • Distracting activities • Protecting and monitoring
Instrumental Support	*Instrumental Support*
• Assistance with material aid or finances and household tasks • Borrowing or loaning of money	• Offers of prayers • Assistance to maintain social roles • Assistance to maintain religious practices • Assistance to remain in the home
Informational Support	*Informational Support*
• Information available from educational programs • Information available from support groups • Information received from healthcare providers	• Getting information about what to expect • Validating information received from health-care providers • Assistance to understand information from healthcare providers

Once I analyzed the data and identified the categories of social support relevant to African American cancer survivors, I returned to the health sciences literature. The purpose of this review was to merge the categories of social support that emerged from the interviews with African Americans with those existing in the larger body of literature. I also returned to the literature in anthropology and history to explain my interpretation of these new categories within the context of what is known in these disciplines about the lived experiences of African Americans and the social support used during adverse situations, see Table 4.2.

Equity and Social Exchange Theories to Understand Reciprocal Supportive Relationships

Social exchange theory was useful in this project to understand ways in which African Americans understand social support. In the healthcare literature, investigators have primarily conceptualized reciprocal relationships as primarily occurring when (1) an equal number of resources are given and received and (2) the exchange is between two persons who know each other (Goodenow et al., 1990; Griffith, 1985; McFarlane et al., 1981; Silverstein & Waite, 1993; Wentowski, 1981).

Studies on reciprocity in social relationships have generally been guided by *equity and social exchange theory*. According to *equity theory*, individuals attempt to maintain fairness and equity in relationships through individual evaluations of what is received in proportion to what is given. Groups attempt to maintain equity in relationships by sharing resources and through evaluations of what each member contributes to the group (Walster et al., 1978). Equity theorists also suggest that when given a choice, individuals attempt to receive more than they give in social relationships (Walster et al., 1978). However, when either too much or too little is received from social relationships, people will attempt to restore equity in those relationships, or they end them.

The *social exchange theory* is also used to explain reciprocity in social relationships. According to social exchange theory, people give or help others with the expectation that their behavior will be rewarded (Homans, 1974). In order to maintain relationships or continue receiving the help of others, people must repay or reciprocate the help or resources they receive. In the next sections, I will introduce ways in which these theories guided the exploration of social relationships that occurred among the women and men studied.

Exchanges in Dyadic Relationships

Two kinds of reciprocal exchanges occurred in a dyadic relationship (two persons) over a short period of time. One occurred when the cancer patient was involved in giving and receiving help over a short period of time. An example was when two close friends, both diagnosed with cancer, were involved in a continual mutual exchange of emotional support. This relationship would be considered reciprocal or balanced since it involved exchanging a resource of equal value between the same two persons (Goodenow et al., 1990; Griffith, 1985; McFarlane et al., 1981). In this study, one example of this type of supportive relationship was in an exchange between two individuals where one survivor received the support of advice and information and paid that support back to the second cancer survivor with emotional support.

A second type of dyadic social relationship was long term and occurred during interactions that led to a new friendship. In these social relationships, the reciprocal exchange was deferred but still expected. In this study, a long-term dyadic supportive relationship when one survivor gave a form of social support to a second survivor. The second survivor reciprocated that support to the first survivor at a later date. In contrast to short-term relationships, deferred exchanges that occurred in dyadic relationships often included the instrument support of a personal service. This type of exchange has also been described as a generalized exchange; these were the norm among persons in established long-term relationships. Help was given with no specified time for repayment. Generalized exchanges also have no agreed upon amount or kind of repayment. Giving in these two-person relationships was based on a trust that when repayment was needed, it would be received.

Exchanges in Group Relationships (Three or More Individuals)

In contrast to those reciprocal relationships that occurred between two persons, a second variation occurred when resources were exchanged among three or more persons. This type of reciprocal exchange occurred when the cancer patient received help from one or more network members that was later paid back to a different network member. In this study, exchanges of social support occurred among three or more persons with no specified time or amount of repayment. Reciprocity between these persons was based on giving to someone in need when a resource was available.

The exchange of social support among group relationships captures the system of mutual aid that has existed among African American communities for generations. This mutual exchange system was a necessary component for the economic survival of African Americans, many of whom lived with incomes below poverty levels. The assumed cultural rule for this exchange was that network members would share available resources with those in the community who were in need. And, although reciprocal exchanges may

have been "imbalanced" at times, individuals remained in this network for the benefit of sharing resources that enabled them to survive.

Theory of Support Bank

The concept of reciprocal exchanges in which social resources are given and received, exchanges governed by what is available and what is needed, is similar to the Support Bank Theory (Antonucci & Jackson, 1990). When individuals are engaged in an exchange system such as a Support Bank, they consciously or unconsciously keep mental records of what they have given and received from this bank over the years. The help and support given are seen as deposits in this Support Bank. When withdrawals are made, or help is received, there is no need to reciprocate since deposits have previously been made into this Support Bank. The theory of a Support Bank for making deposits and withdrawals of resources is grounded in several theoretical papers. In one, Gouldner (1960) stated that engaging in reciprocal relationships is a learned behavior. According to Gouldner (1960) people learn that helping others is a criterion for receiving help. This statement supports an expression from one participant who said "in order to receive help you must have given help."

The theory of a Support Bank enables one to understand that reciprocal relationships occur among individuals known to one another but is inclusive of strangers. This occurs since anyone can make deposits or withdrawals with the Support Bank. With a Support Bank, reciprocal relationships occur when help is received from one person but paid back to another person with whom there has been no previous relationship. In this study, the cancer patient received help during the treatment phase of the cancer trajectory and later gave help back to other cancer patients during their treatment phase.

The findings that emerged using the theory of a Support Bank expanded our understanding of the exchange of social support that occurs among African American cancer survivors. Prior to this research, support during cancer was believed to primarily come from family and friends. However, our findings show that when there is a perceived Support Bank, social support is exchanged among a broader network of individuals known to the cancer patient but from individuals who are basically strangers.

There are two possible explanations for helping relative strangers. One explanation is that this form of helping is a form of altruism (Gouldner, 1960; Leeds, 1963; Zabielski, 1984). According to Leeds (1963), acts of giving are altruistic when they are voluntary and not in response to role obligations and when the intended action is to "do good." Relationships among the cancer patients in this study were indeed volunteered—hence the response from one participant for others to "call me if you need me." The intended purpose of the relationships was to do a good deed and was not in response to any specified family or work obligations. The cancer patients helping each other had no established relationships; they were introduced through friends or relatives. Moreover, no effort was made to maintain the relationships. The reward to the giver was intrinsic: feelings of satisfaction from helping someone.

A second explanation was that these acts of helping were efforts to pay back the help received from someone else (Berkowitz & Daniels, 1964; Leeds, 1963; Zabielski, 1984). In this study, cancer patients who received help from others during the treatment phase of their cancer trajectory likely felt an obligation to return that help to other cancer patients. The finding of acts of altruism among African Americans is not surprising, especially given their social history. Historical accounts contain many examples of acts of altruism as African Americans participated in service-oriented clubs and organizations developed for the primary purpose of helping those less fortunate (Du Bois, 1978; Giddings, 1984; Lerner, 1979; Powdermaker, 1937/1993). Sociologist Andrew Billingsley (1992) gives an example of how altruistic giving can inspire recipients to pay back others. He tells the story of a student who received money to help pay college tuition from a teacher who wanted her to complete her education. This student completed college and became successfully employed. However, rather than pay back the money received from the teacher, she repaid the debt by helping other struggling students.

A third explanation for this perception of a Support Bank is likely grounded in the strong religious culture of African Americans. Religious scholars suggest that altruistic giving is grounded in religious doctrines (Wilmore, 2000). According to Wilmore (2000) one such doctrine is that as God's children, we are expected to "lift as we climb" (Wilmore, 2000). Wilmore (2000) argues that "lifting as we climb" is a religious doctrine accepted by African Americans that comes from the old spiritual, "Climbing Jacobs Ladder." The lyrics of this spiritual give meaning to climbing upward out of misery and suffering toward a God that called for them to be "soldiers of the cross." Being soldiers of the cross dictated a life of self-improvement but also lending a hand to help anyone who needs help. Rewards for this type of giving come not from the receiver but later in the form of eternal life in Heaven.

Several religious doctrines from the Bible are used to support reciprocal exchanges of giving first and receiving later. One example comes from the sixth chapter of Galatians. These verses stipulate that in order to receive help when needed and benefit from eternal life in heaven, "one must help others at every opportunity." Another widely held doctrine from the Bible, also in Galatians, proclaims "You shall reap what you sow." This verse has commonly been translated to mean "if you give, you will also receive." An implicit meaning in this verse is that future receiving will be determined by present giving. Individuals accepting these doctrines are motivated to help others in the belief that as givers they will benefit at a later time.

Example 2. Faith-Based Storytelling Intervention

The overwhelming uses of theory in the qualitative projects I have conducted have been explicitly stated and used to guide the study design, sampling strategies, data collection and analysis of projects. This next exemplar study supported the development of an intervention to alleviate psychological distress through a series of positive stories about cancer, suggesting that cancer is not a death sentence. In fact, the goal of this exemplar study was to enable African American cancer patients to see individuals similar to them, living well after a cancer diagnosis and treatment. The greater impact of this intervention was to decrease mental suffering and assist the African American cancer patient and their family members in their attempt to engage in supportive relationships during the diagnosis and treatment of cancer.

The development of the *Faith-based Intervention* was guided by Stress and Coping and Transportation Theories and used a combination of quantitative and qualitative research designs. The aims of this feasibility study were to develop and evaluate the usability and acceptability of the *Faith-Based African American Cancer Survivorship Storytelling Intervention*. Consider the quote from a cancer family member below in support of this storytelling intervention. This quote illustrates the stigma that persists in the African American community regarding cancer.

> "I think that's put out there, you know automatically the stigma that cancer is death...It would have been helpful to hear somebody say, my mother had the same situation and she's fine, she still looks like herself. She's not different, she's healthy, and she's beating cancer. That would have been helpful, because a lot of times that is opposite of what you hear. If you only hear the negative, she's gonna lose weight, she's gonna lose her hair, a lot of times people don't make it, and they die...but if you hear positive things... it will be real beneficial. I feel like my outlook would have been stronger, I probably would have went to more appointments, [been] more supportive and able to encourage her."

The first aim of this study was the development of the intervention using a series of professionally edited narrative video recordings. The recordings were of African American cancer patient and family caregiver survivorship narratives that were grounded in the strong religious culture of African Americans. These stories were captured during the conduct of a qualitative research project using a qualitative descriptive design that was guided by the research question "What are the strategies used among African American Cancer Survivors in response to a cancer diagnosis?" The use of this abstract research question permitted the African American cancer survivors to give voice to strategies important to their experiences. The collection of stories was coded by expert reviewers with member checking by the target population to identify themes in these stories. Concepts from Stress and Coping Theory were used to carefully select video-recorded narratives to capture the essence of cancer patients and family caregivers describing the stressors encountered, strategies used in response to the distress experienced, and their perceived mental health outcomes from the use of these strategies. This selection of video-recorded stories was professionally edited by a multi-media expert with oversight from the research team.

The second aim of this study was to understand usability and acceptability of this intervention through the narratives of participants. For this aim, usability was evaluated through participants' perceived clarity, persuasiveness, and ease of use. Acceptability was evaluated through enrollment, participation, and concepts of Transportation Theory (identification, engagement, and emotional response). In the next sections, I describe in detail the use of Stress and Coping Theory to guide the construction of the stories and the use of Transportation Theory to guide the qualitative evaluation of usability and acceptability of the intervention.

Stress and Coping Theoretical Framework. The development of the *Faith-Based African American Cancer Survivorship Stories Intervention* was guided by concepts in Stress and Coping Theory (Green & Brock, 2000; Murphy et al., 2013). Stress and Coping theory has been used to examine mental health promoting strategies among African American cancer patients (Hamilton et al., 2009; Northouse et al., 2010). According to this theory, when an event is perceived as stressful, individuals use strategies to affect the stressor or to change the perception of the stressor (Lazarus & Folkman, 1984). Among African Americans, social support has been a dominant strategy to change the perceived threat of cancer as an emotion-focused strategy (Hamilton et al., 2007; Holt et al., 2012). For this intervention, Stress and Coping theory has guided the selection of stories wherein the narrator articulates a beginning (stressful event), middle (social support as a coping strategy), and end (mental health outcome).

Transportation Theory (TT). Transportaton Theory (TT) has been useful in examining the influences of narratives on health promoting behavior change among African Americans (Goddu et al., 2015; Houston et al., 2011; Murphy et al., 2013), to promote cancer screening behaviors (Ellis et al., 2018; Kreuter et al., 2010; McQueen et al., 2011) and adherence to cancer follow-up care (Perez et al., 2014). TT posits that a change in attitudes and behaviors is enhanced through the identification and emotional engagement of a viewer with the narrative. Therefore, the selection of stories incorporated into this intervention considers: (1) similarity to and identification with narrators in the recordings; and (2) the emotional engagement of participants with selected recordings. We specifically organized interview questions to capture the following:

Acceptability. How interesting were the video-recorded stories?

Usability. How easy (or difficult) was it to access the stories? Were the Stories too long (not long enough)? Was the content applicable to your situation? Did the stories persuade you to change your attitude or perspective toward cancer?

Identification with Storyteller. Where storytellers in the videos likeable? Which storytellers did you identify with?

Narrative Engagement with Stories. Did you have any expectations when you were watching the video-recorded stories, did videos grab and hold your attention?

Emotional Response to the Stories. Did any of the stories bring about any emotions such as hopefulness, anger, sadness, anxiety?

Using these combined frameworks of Stress and Coping and Transportation Theories, the final selection of recordings for the intervention consists of those stories most likely to influence positive affective (decrease psychological distress) and behavioral changes (engage in supportive social networks) among the targeted population.

Our preliminary findings suggest that the *Faith-based African American Cancer Survivorship Stories Intervention* was emotionally engaging for the study participants since storytelling is an important aspect of the cultural history of this population. Although storytelling is familiar to this population, when faced with a new and very distressful situation such as cancer, assistance is needed to rethink and reconceptualize this very important aspect of their cultural foundation. Consider the following quotes from participants after they had viewed the series of video-recorded stories that captured *Usability and Acceptability* as well as the concepts in Transportation Theory: *Identification, Narrative Engagement with the stories, and Emotional Response to the stories:*

Acceptability. "The videos give you the motivation to go out and talk to your friends and your family and try to help them [be more accepting of the diagnosis]."

Usability. "I hate to say they're too short but they're so good. You only get a little bit of them. For me, I could probably do this all day long, go home feeling so much better. I'm glad we did this now."

Identification with Storyteller. "And that one guy, I could relate to him. I mean cause like I said, his story was my story. It seemed like he was talking about me and he don't even know me. Word for word, I was pretty much going to say the same things he was saying. And that really connected with me and it's more people like me that sharing their stories and they got their testaments they putting out there."

Narrative Engagement with Stories. "The one lady with the blonde hair that sung 'I Won't Complain'. I like her the best. She looked healthy. She looked like when she sang her song like she kinda was giving a testimony."

Emotional Response to the Stories. "I felt happy or sad when the characters in the story were happy or sad… I felt happy a lot…I could feel the emotions of some of the characters in the story."

Paradigms/Theories in Qualitative Research

There are paradigms/theories that have historically influenced or shaped the qualitative researcher's approach or perspective to a project. These have included *Post Positivism, Critical Theory/Critical Race Theory, Feminist Theory, and Intersectionality*. In this section, I will describe briefly these with ways these paradigms and/or theories have influenced my perceptions of social support as an SDOH among African American populations.

Postpositivist. Scholars embracing this traditional perspective of science believe multiple realities exist and integrate multiple levels of rigor/validity into the research process (Denzin & Lincoln, 2012). Postpositivist values the traditional scientific method while recognizing that science is not truly objective but that conclusions are influenced by experiences and biases of the researcher. As an African American scholar, I frequently argued against the postpositivist perspective and the limitation that knowledge generated about African American populations has been and continues to be through the lens of white and middle-class scientists. This postpositivist perspective drives a research process that largely is developed in isolation of the community and ignores the voices of minority populations. There may also be a perspective and devaluing among the majority group of scientists that evidence generated by African Americans studying African Americans as too subjective. I frequently argue that all science is subjective, with majority of scientists deciding what research questions are important and relevant, what methods are best suited to answer the questions, the use of measures that are typically developed and validated with white populations, to the interpretation of findings generated among research teams that exclude members of the target population or other scientists of color.

Critical Theory/Critical Race Theory. Critical Theory is the perspective that power structures and inequalities that exist among social systems are oppressive to minority populations (Held, 1980). Scholars embracing *Critical Theory* would challenge the status quo to consider power imbalances in the care delivered to oppressed and marginal populations such as African Americans. For example, rather than placing the blame for the increased advanced staging of cancer on the patient, the scholar of *Critical Theory* would emphasize the inequities in income, education, insured status, and lack of access to care as factors that should be considered. *Critical Race Theory*. Generally recognized as an educational framework, *Critical Race Theory* has been met with increased scrutiny and debate. According to this framework, racism is embedded throughout educational and healthcare institutions and legal systems (Crenshaw et al., 1996). As such, racism is inherent in our laws, policies, and influences the care delivered to minority populations. Scholars who explore healthcare issues through a Critical Race Theory perspective would argue that the practice of examining race in research ignores that race is a biological construct and should not be used as an attributing factor to health outcomes. Rather than race, the influencing factor to health disparities and health inequalities is the individual experience with racism.

Feminist Theory. This is an approach to science that considers the ways in which gender shapes the illness experience and influences of the social determinants of health. According to Feminist Theory women, particularly African American women, have historically been oppressed, marginalized, and disadvantaged (Collins, 1991). Social support theories in existence today originated from research on the social support used and available to males in organizational settings during the 1970s (Kahn & Antonucci, 1980). This research focused on the role-expectations and resources of male executives in the workplace (Kahn & Antonucci, 1980). The findings indicated that work-related stressors were buffered by the social support received from supervisors, colleagues, and subordinates. Findings from these earlier studies with white men suggested that low amounts of social support were attributed to poor relations with coworkers and decreased resources from supervisors that resulted in an inability to perform work roles, and from a health perspective, they had higher risk factors associated with heart disease, high blood pressure, and serum glucose levels (Kahn & Antonucci, 1980). This research was important for validating the received aspect of social support on health outcomes and well-being. However, conceptualizations of social support in this earlier research excluded the voices of African American women who have occupied a subordinate status in this country while tending to give or provide support to assist others in the achievement of their goals (Levitt et al., 1985).

Intersectionality Theory. Although this framework began with the inclusion of influence of social identities related to race, gender, and class, *Intersectionality Theory* has expanded into a lens for understanding how individual social, cultural, and political identities are interwoven to influence health outcomes (Collins, 2019; Crenshaw, 2017). Intersectionality Theory influences a perspective that individuals have multiple intersecting identities (like race, ethnicity, religion, gender, class, ability, sexual orientation, etc.) that influence their lived experiences and response to illness situations. Further, researchers guided by *Intersectionality Theory* recognize that individual identities do not operate in a vacuum but integrated and overlapping. For example, a Black woman's illness experience is shaped by her gender but also her racial identity, culture, religious identity, and class—these are not separate factors but rather interwoven aspects of her identity.

Conclusion

The use of theory in qualitative research is critical to ensure a rigorous project throughout study design, sampling, data collection, and data analysis. In this chapter, I have illustrated with two exemplar studies ways in which theory emerged from the findings of a qualitative research project and ways in which theory guided the revision of a construct in a qualitative project. The goal of this chapter was to showcase that theory is used to guide research that aims to explain associations, test hypotheses, or predict outcomes in intervention studies. On the other hand, theory in qualitative research is used as a lens to understand a phenomenon or meanings derived from individual lived experiences. I have also included a discussion of when and how to use a review of the literature and ways in which I have reviewed the health sciences literature iteratively. For example, a review of the literature can be used to identify the gaps prior to conducting projects, during the interviews to better understand emerging themes, while interpreting data collected, and to explain the findings in the discussion sections of manuscripts. I have also described how I move from a review of the literature in the health sciences to a review of the literature in other disciplines as needed. This expanded review assists with generating information-rich cases and a final project that is enriching for all.

References

Antonucci, T. C. and J. S. Jackson (1990). The role of reciprocity in social support. *Social Support: An Interactional View*. B. R. Sarason, G. Irwin, G. Sarason and G. R. Pierce (Eds.). New York, John Wiley & Sons: 173–198.

Berkowitz, L. and L. R. Daniels (1964). "Effects of past help on the response to dependency relationships." *J Abnorm Soc Psychol* **68**(3): 275–281.

Billingsley, A. (1992). *Climbing Jacob's Ladder: The Enduring Legacy of African-American Families*. New York, Simon & Schuster.

Chatters, L. M., R. J. Taylor and R. Jayakody (1994). "Fictive kinship relations in black extended families." *J Comp Fam Stud* **25**(3): 297–312.

Collins, P. H. (1991). *Black Feminist Thought*. New York, Routledge, Chapman and Hall, Inc.

Collins, P. H. (2019). *Interesctionality: As Critical Social Theory*. Durham and London, Duke University Press.

Crenshaw, K. W. (2017). *On Intersectionality: Essential Writings*. New York, The New Press.

Crenshaw, K. W., N. Gotanda and G. Peller. (1996). *Critical Race Theory: The Key Writings That Formed the Movement*. New York, The New Press.

Degazon, C. E. (1994). "Ethnic identification, social support and coping strategies among three groups of ethnic African elders." *J Cult Divers* **1**(4): 79–85.

Denzin, N. K. and Y. S. Lincoln. (2012). *The Landscape of Qualitative Research*. Thousand Oaks, CA, Sage Publishing.

Du Bois, W. E. B. (1978). *On Sociology and the Black community*. Chicago, Ill, University of Chicago Press.

Ellis, E. M., D. O. Erwin, L. Jandorf, F. Saad-Harfouche, P. Sriphanlop, N. Clark, C. Dauphin, D. Johnson, L. B. Klasko-Foster, C. Martinez, J. Sly, D. White, G. Winkel and M. T. Kiviniemi. (2018). "Designing a randomized controlled trial to evaluate a community-based narrative intervention for improving colorectal cancer screening for African Americans." *Contemp Clin Trials* **65**: 8–18.

Ellison, C. G. (1995). "Race, religious involvement and depressive symptomatology in a southeastern U.S. community." *Soc Sci Med* **40**(11): 1561–1572.

Giddings, P. (1984). *When and Where I Enter: The Impact of Black Women on Race and Sex in America*. New York, William Morrow.

Goddu, A. P., K. E. Raffel and M. E. Peek. (2015). "A story of change: The influence of narrative on African-Americans with diabetes." *Patient Educ Couns* **98**(8): 1017–1024.

Goodenow C, S. T. Reisine and K E. Grady (1990). "Quality of social support and associated social and psychological functioning in women with rheumatoid arthritis." *Health Psychol* **9**(3): 266–284. doi: 10.1037//0278-6133.9.3.266.

Gouldner, A. W. (1960). The norm of reciprocity: A preliminary statement. *Am Sociol Rev* **25**(2): 161–178.

Griffith, J. (1985). "Social support providers: Who are they? Where are they met? and the relationship of network characteristics to psychological distress." *Basic Appl Soc Psychol* **6**(1): 41–60.

Green, M. C. and T. C. Brock. (2000). "The role of transportation in the persuasiveness of public narratives." *J Pers Soc Psychol* **79**(5): 701–721.

Hamilton, J., B. Powe, A. Pollard, K. Lee and A. Felton. (2007). "Spirituality among African American cancer survivors." *Cancer Nurs* **30**(3): 309–316.

Hamilton, J. B., B. J. Stewart, J. L. Crandell and M. R. Lynn. (2009). "Development of the ways of helping questionnaire: A measure of preferred coping strategies for older African American cancer survivors." *Res Nurs Health* **32**(3): 243–259.

Helgeson, V. S. and S. Cohen, (1996). "Social support and adjustment to cancer: Reconciling descriptive, correlational, and intervention research." *Health Psychol* **15**(2): 135–148.

Held, D. (1980). *Introduction to Critical Theory*. Berkeley, CA, University of California Press.

Holt, C. L., E. Schulz, L. Caplan, V. Blake, V. L. Southward and A. V. Buckner. (2012). "Assessing the role of spirituality in coping among African Americans diagnosed with cancer." *J Relig Health* **51**(2): 507–521.

Homans, G. C. (1974). *Social Behavior: Its Elementary Forms*. New York, Harcourt Publishers.

House, J. S. and R. L. Kahn, (1985). Measures and concepts of social support. In S. Cohen, & S. L. Syme (Eds.), *Social Support and Health*. Orlando, FL, Academic Press: 83–108.

Houston, T. K., J. J. Allison, M. Sussman, W. Horn, C. L. Holt, J. Trobaugh, M. Salas, M. Pisu, Y. L. Cuffee, D. Larkin, S. D. Person, B. Barton, C. I. Kiefe and S. Hullett. (2011). "Culturally appropriate storytelling to improve blood pressure: A randomized trial." *Ann Intern Med* **154**(2): 77–84.

Jayakody, R., L. Chatters and R. J Taylor (1993). "Family support to single and married African American mothers: The provision of financial, emotional, and child care assistance." *J Marriage Fam* **55**: 261–276.

Kahn, R. L. and T. C. Antonucci (1980). Convoys Over the Life Course: Attachment, Roles, and Social Support. *Life-Span Development and Behavior*. P. B. Baltes and O. G. Grim. New York, Academic Press. **3**: 253–286.

Kreuter, M. W., K. Holmes, K. Alcaraz, B. Kalesan, S. Rath, M. Richert, A. McQueen, N. Caito, L. Robinson and E. M. Clark. (2010). "Comparing narrative and informational videos to increase mammography in low-income African American women." *Patient Educ Couns* **81**: S6–14.

Lazarus, R. S. and S. Folkman. (1984). *Stress, Appraisal, and Coping*. New York, Springer Publishing Company.

Leeds, R. (1963). Altruism and the norm of giving. *Merrill-Palmer* **9**(3): *Q* 229–240.

Lerner, G. (1979). *The Majority Finds Its Past: Placing Women in History*. New York, Oxford University Press.

Levitt, M. J., T. C. Antonucci, M. C. Clark, J. Rotton and G. E. Finley. (1985). "Social support and well-being: Preliminary indicators based on two samples of the elderly." *Int J Aging Hum Dev* **21**(1): 61–77.

McFarlane, A. H., K. A. Neale, G. R. Norman, R. G. Roy and D. L. Streiner (1981). "Methodological issues in developing a scale to measure social support." *Schizophr Bull* **7**(1): 90–100.

McQueen, A., M. W. Kreuter, B. Kalesan and K. I. Alcaraz. (2011). "Understanding narrative effects: The impact of breast cancer survivor stories on message processing, attitudes, and beliefs among African American women." *Health Psychol* **30**(6): 674–682.

Murphy, S. T., L. B. Frank, J. S. Chatterjee and L. Baezconde-Garbanati. (2013). "Narrative versus non-narrative: The role of identification, transportation and emotion in reducing health disparities." *J Commun* **63**: 1–19).

Northouse, L. L., M. C. Katapodi, L. Song, L. Zhang and D. W. Mood. (2010). "Interventions with family caregivers of cancer patients: Meta-analysis of randomized trials." *CA Cancer J Clin* **60**(5): 317–39.

Perez, M., J. A. Sefko, D. Ksiazek, B. Golla, C. Casey, J. A. Margenthaler, G. Colditz, M. W. Kreuter and D. B. Jeffe. (2014). "A novel intervention using interactive technology and personal narratives to reduce cancer disparities: African American breast cancer survivor stories." *J Cancer Surviv* **8**(1): 21–30.

Powdermaker, H. (1937–1993). *After Freedom: A Cultural Study in the Deep South*. Madison, WS, University of Wisconsin Press.

Silverstein M. and L. J. Waite (1993). "Are blacks more likely than whites to receive and provide social support in middle and old age? Yes, no, and maybe so." *J Gerontol* **48**(4): S212–S222. doi: 10.1093/geronj/48.4.s212.

Tilden, V. P. (1985). "Issues of conceptualization and measurement of social support in the construction of nursing theory." *Res Nurs Health* **8**: 199–206.

Walster, E., G. W. Walster and E. Berscheid (1978). *Equity: Theory and Research*. Boston, MA: Allyn and Bacon.

Wentowski, G. J. (1981). Reciprocity and the coping strategies of older people: Cultural dimensions of network building. *Gerontologist*, **21**(6): 600–609.

Wilmore, G. S. (2000). *Black Religion and Black Radicalism*. Maryknoll, NY, Orbis Books.

Zabielski, M. T. (1984). Giving and receiving in the neomaternal period: A case of distributive inequity. *Matern Child Nurs J* **13**(1): 19–46.

5 Sampling Strategies for SDOH Topics in Community Engaged Research

Gaining access to underrepresented communities is an extremely time-intensive process. It can take years, literally, to develop trusting, collaborative relationships in any community. In this chapter, I describe my beginnings accessing community-dwelling African American populations and the sampling strategies used throughout my career to recruit and enroll this population into qualitative research projects. This chapter consists of two sections:

1 How to identify target populations for SDOH research in underrepresented communities

- The location and recruitment of participants in community purposive sampling (convenient, criterion, maximum variation, theoretical, snowball)
- Exemplars of recruitment and enrollment of appropriate participants in underrepresented communities

2 Critical examination of determinations of sample size (saturation, informational redundancy)

- Theoretical saturation
- Data Saturation/informational redundancy

Purposeful Sampling with Criterion and Maximum Variation

My first research experience using qualitative methods was with my dissertation project.

Through my mentors, Merle Mishel, PhD, RN, FAAN, and Barbara Germino, PhD, RN, FAAN, I had access to participants from three larger federally funded studies, two awarded to PI Merle Mishel, RN, PhD, FAAN, and one to Carrie Braden, RN, PhD, FAAN. The aim of these studies was to test a psycho-educational intervention delivered to underserved women being treated for breast cancer and men treated for localized prostate cancer.

I initially recruited and interviewed a convenient sample of African American women with breast cancer from lists of participants of completed NIH-funded research projects. These African American women were sampled from the Managing Uncertainty: Self-Help in Breast Cancer funded to PI Merle Mishel, PhD, RN, FAAN, and Promoting Self-Help: Underserved Women with Breast Cancer funded to PI Carrie Braden, PhD, RN, FAAN. The Managing Uncertainty in Breast Cancer Studies were designed to deliver a psycho-educational intervention to underserved African American, Caucasian, and Mexican

DOI: 10.4324/9781003598916-5

American women being treated for breast cancer. The primary purpose of these studies was to help these women increase their knowledge of breast cancer, and enhance self-help, and self-care behaviors through a telephone intervention delivered by nurses. The intervention was delivered during the treatment phase of their illness with the overall goal of improving quality of life for these women.

After interviewing the women, I was given access to a list for African American men that had completed an uncertainty intervention for men diagnosed with prostate cancer. This was a wonderful opportunity given that over 25 years ago, African American men were an understudied population, and few NIH studies were funded to conduct research with this specific patient population. The African American men recruited were from a third federally funded study, the Managing Uncertainty in Stage B Prostate Cancer funded to PI Merle Mishel, RN, PhD, FAAN. The primary study was an uncertainty management intervention delivered to African American and Caucasian men with stage B or early-stage C prostate cancer and recruited either after surgical treatment or during the early phase of radiation therapy. A family member, usually a spouse, was also recruited into the study. The purpose of this study was to improve symptom control, uncertainty management, and psychosocial functioning in men with localized prostate cancer. These participant lists were a convenient sample that was necessary to access the target population during the early phase of my research career. I had limited resources and was under a time constraint to complete the study during my doctoral studies.

In the sections below, I describe ways in which I incorporated types of purposeful sampling to recruit African American women and men into my qualitative research project. Purposeful sampling is a sampling strategy associated with qualitative research and is a recruitment process where participants are deliberately selected based on a specific characteristic. Participants are purposefully identified as those most appropriate to provide information rich information on the topic of interest (Maxwell, 2013; Merriam & Tisdell, 2016). Other types of purposeful sampling include criterion, maximum variation, and theoretical. Criterion sampling is simply the identification of participants based on a selected criteria which in this study was the self-identification of being African American and having a diagnosis of breast or prostate cancer. Maximum variation was another type of purposeful sampling added to ensure a diverse population of cancer survivors to capture a range of social support experiences in response to a cancer diagnosis (Maxwell, 2013; Merriam & Tisdell, 2016). A third, theoretical sampling, is done during the process of data collection to select participants based on questions that emerge from the data. Unlike the other types of purposeful sampling, theoretical sampling cannot be determined prior to a study and is generally used with the grounded theory approach (Maxwell, 2013; Merriam & Tisdell, 2016). Finally, snowball sampling is also sometimes viewed as a form of purposeful sampling. This approach to recruitment can be beneficial when attempting to gain entry into a new and unfamiliar community, and the researcher could benefit from referrals to other participants.

Criterion sampling of cancer survivors who had completed treatment. In this section, I describe my experience with criterion sampling as a type of purposeful sampling to recruit African American women and men with the experience of having had a cancer diagnosis and completed treatment. I specifically selected this patient population for their expertise with accessing social support during the diagnosis and treatment for cancer. The participants I recruited for my qualitative project were drawn from the previously described population of cancer survivors. For recruitment of participants for my research, I was given access to a list of African American women and men who had completed the intervention and final data collection phase of the larger studies. Given this list, I sent out a mailing to recruit participants for my qualitative project on social support among African American cancer patients. The mailing was a one-page letter with my picture a brief bio and brief description of the research project I was proposing. Participants were given a stamped, self-addressed envelope should they not want to be contacted by phone. After a one-to-two-week period, I made phone calls to participants I had mailed and those who had not opted out.

Maximum variation for heterogeneity and transferability. In this same study, I also used another type of purposeful sampling which was maximum variation (Maxwell, 2013; Merriam & Tisdell, 2016). Using maximum variation, I deliberately varied the selection of African American women and men according to key variables identified as being important from the social support literature. Among these variables were gender, age, marital status, income, education, geographic region, and proximity to family (Kahn & Antonucci, 1980). However, due to restrictions imposed when sampling from an available list of participants, I was only able to select women and men that varied on gender, marital status, educational level, geographic location, and proximity to family.

African American women and men were recruited for this study to capture the influence of gender on the experience of social support. Findings from some studies suggest differences in the structure of network members between African American women and men (Brown & Gary, 1987). For example, while African American women turn to other female friends and relatives in response to female-related health problems (Mathews et al., 1994), African American men turn to brothers and fathers in response to the stresses of serious problems (Broman, 1991; Taylor et al., 1996).

Other studies indicate differences among women and men in the social support that is available and used in response to stress (Broman, 1991; Chatters et al., 1994). The few studies on social support among African Americans suggest that African American women may be more actively involved in providing social support to others. In research with African American males and females with a variety of health problems, Brown & Gary (1987) found that the women in this study tended to give more support than they received. In other studies, it is the African American woman who is most active in providing childcare and advice to others with health problems (Neighbors & Howard, 1987; Neighbors & Jackson, 1984).

Although there are gender differences in social network structure and patterns of providing social support, the historical influences of racism, oppression, and limited external resources have influenced similar responses to problems. For example, both African American women and men have been active participants in a mutual system of sharing resources (Jones, 1995). African American women and men are also active providers of social support as members of organized church groups (Powdermaker, 1937/1993; Lincoln, 1974) and extended families (Chatters et al., 1994; Dressler, 1985).

The second decision was to identify African American women and men who varied on marital status. The larger body of social support literature informs us that the spouse is the most important source of social support. However, this finding is the result of sampling white, middle class, and married persons. In comparison, the literature on social support among African Americans suggests that extended families, rather than spouses, are the most important source of support for this population. When it comes to the amount of social support provided to married and unmarried persons, investigators have found that extended family members are actively involved in providing social support regardless of marital status (Brown & Gary, 1985; Hatch, 1991). In fact, the amount of social support provided to unmarried persons from extended family members has exceeded that provided to married persons (Brown & Gary, 1985; Jayakody et al., 1993). There are no studies that specifically examine the types of social support provided to married and unmarried African Americans experiencing chronic and life-threatening health problems.

The third decision was to recruit African American men and women from different educational backgrounds. Among Caucasian persons, levels of education influence both social network size and social support (Mathews et al., 1994; Primomo et al., 1990). For example, many researchers have found that those persons with higher levels of education also tend to be more actively involved in group and church activities and to also receive more social support (Mathews et al., 1994; Primomo et al., 1990). For African Americans, with the exception of examinations of educational level on size of social networks (Chatters et al., 1994) and amounts of social support provided to a healthy, elderly population (Walls, 1992), there have been no studies that directly address the influence of educational levels on social support among chronically ill members of this population.

A fourth sampling procedure was to recruit African American men and women from urban and rural areas. Although the men and women participating in these interviews reside in North Carolina, I attempted to vary the participants according to areas recognized as metropolitan areas and those recognized as townships. According to social support studies among African American populations, geographic location does influence size and durability of social networks. African Americans residing in more rural areas are more likely to have long-standing relationships among family and friends, and persons residing in the South are more likely to have more extensive social networks (Chatters et al., 1994).

A final maximum variation sampling procedure was to recruit African American women and men according to proximity of family members. Social support researchers frequently obtain information on the proximity of individuals to their social networks. However, few investigators have attempted to directly link proximity of network members to other variables. African Americans living in southern and rural areas tend to report higher numbers of family members and relatives living close by (Chatters et al., 1994). Additionally, the support from extended family to residents living in close proximity in a Southern community resulted in their having fewer symptoms of depression (Dressler, 1985).

In social support research, close proximity has been defined as those persons living within a few miles of individuals needing social support. In this study, being in close proximity was defined as living within the same household. Therefore, participants were selected based on whether they lived with someone or lived alone.

I conducted all of the interviews in the participants' homes. This setting was selected for the participants' convenience and also because I believed being in a familiar environment would reduce any anxiety from discussing personal issues with a stranger. Participants did speak candidly and freely about their experiences with the cancer diagnosis and treatment but also about their experiences with social support. Some participants had family members present during the interviews, while some participants scheduled the interviews when family members would be away. Interviews lasted from 45 minutes to 2 hours and were conducted until informational redundancy or theoretical saturation was achieved within the key variables selected (Strauss & Corbin, 1998). That is, until no new concepts related to social support emerged from the data.

Purposeful Sampling with Criterion and Theoretical Sampling

A second exemplar study, *Perceptions of Support among Older African American Cancer Survivors,* illustrates the purposeful sampling of theoretical sampling with a grounded theory qualitative approach (Hamilton et al., 2010). The purpose of this study was to explore the perceived needs for social support for African American cancer survivors. Grounded theory techniques of theoretical sampling and constant comparison (to be described in the data analysis chapter) were used for the purpose of typology development (Strauss, 1999). Theoretical sampling consisted of sampling interview data for different manifestations of those factors that influenced participants' social support needs. The authors further examined the data for differences in gender, marital status, education level, and proximity to family. Participants were interviewed until information redundancy and theoretical saturation of emerging themes were achieved (Strauss, 1999).

Theoretical sampling defined selection of participants throughout data collection to inform or refine developing theory. However, in this project, theoretical sampling and constant comparison were used to guide sampling of interview data during data collection for an exploration of topics and questions that emerged during data collection. In the sections to follow, I describe topics that emerged during data collection that I followed up on in each subsequent interview. I have made it a practice now to include in IRB applications that I may need to conduct a second or follow-up interview should additional information be needed.

Receiving support from family and friends. In previous projects, the study goal was to better understand the types of social support provided among networks of family and friends. The questioning in this project that focused on the support needs of African American cancer survivors permitted a look into the types of social support that were forthcoming, as well as those interactions where support was lacking or less desirable. One emerging theme was the expressed disappointment in family members who failed to provide needed support. These participants attributed the fear of death, pain, or suffering that led to family members and friends not showing up to support them or responding with negative or inappropriate comments. Comments below suggested that I need to incorporate interview questions to capture experiences when family and friends were not physically or emotionally available in many ways.

> Now I would like for my husband to have been more supportive. But then I think he was scared. And he wouldn't support me. I could…I still can't talk to him about my cancer.

> …some people don't come around you any more. You know like maybe it's gonna rub off… or something. You know, maybe people just don't wanna be there knowing the fact that you have it. I don't know what it is, but um, I just seen the differences in, in certain people

Another topic that emerged during data collection was the lack of support from church members or when support was forthcoming, it was undesirable and even inappropriate at times. See the quote below:

> I never told my church family. Because I didn't want the pastor standing up there saying, 'Sister B" has…is in the hospital. She has breast cancer. And then everybody oh, poor "J". I did not want that. I…because I had seen how they do others. And as much as I had been promoting breast health education among the African-American I knew some of the things to say and something not to say. So I didn't want him [the Pastor] going up there in the pulpit and people feeling sorry, you know, for me.

This quote led to a sampling of participants who were church members as well as those not affiliated with the Church. Interview questioning considered the participants experience with social support in the church. An example interview question was "Are you a member of a church?" and "What has been your experience with receiving social support from fellow church members?" Whether a church member or not, I still wanted to explore their experiences with individuals who were church members. Was it negative or positive? What were those interactions like?

Purposeful Sampling with Criterion and Snowball Sampling

Probably the experience with snowball sampling in Portland, Oregon is one I will never forget. I had moved to Portland from Durham, North Carolina for a two-year postdoctoral fellowship at Oregon Health & Science University. As an independent academic researcher, I was conducting a pilot study to evaluate a new and culturally relevant measure of social support that captured the strengths of African Americans. It was fall 2001, in my postdoctoral fellowship at OHSU in Portland, Oregon, when I was planning to recruit for this pilot study. I will always remember submitting my application to the University IRB and being initially denied since, based on the reviewer's belief, I would never be able to recruit African American cancer survivors in Portland. Not that my project would cause harm, but I would not be able to recruit this population. Portland was the whitest city I had ever lived, and statistics supported my perception and likely that of this IRB reviewer, since only 2.6% of the population was non-Hispanic, Black. I had traveled across country from Durham, North Carolina and didn't know anyone in Portland except for my two white mentors at Oregon Health & Science University (OHSU). I had joined a Black Church in Portland but had not been there long enough to establish a trusting research collaboration with Portland's Black community.

I pushed back with that IRB reviewer, and eventually received approval to conduct my research, but still had no idea where to start. I distributed flyers in restrooms on campus, flyers in the church bulletin, and flyers in community restaurants. Nothing. However, as luck would have it, I happened to be in the Post Office one afternoon and saw an African American women wearing a T-shirt with the logo "Breast cancer survivor" and a pink ribbon. Being from the South and having previously lived in a city with a large percentage of African Americans, I was glad to see another African American woman and even more excited that she appeared to be a breast cancer survivor. I introduced myself, explained my research on the spot (it is important to have your elevator speech together) and asked if I could interview her. She said yes, I will call you in about two hours when I get home. I gave her my phone number and thought, well I'll never see her again. To my surprise, she called me within two hours, and by the end of the day, she had set me up for interviews with other African American cancer survivors in Northeast Portland. I had tapped into an informal support group of African American cancer survivors in Northeast Portland, and by the month's end, I had interviewed the 30 participants I needed for my pilot study. I was repeatedly told by this group of cancer survivors that they would participate in research at Oregon Health & Science University, but they had never been asked. Portland's Black community was saying, "we would participate in their research, but they never come down off that hill and ask us."

Snowball can be a successful recruitment strategy to get started but researchers may need to consider using an additional sampling strategy should participants fail to provide information-rich data. I was fortunate to have tapped into a population of African American cancer survivors who were truly experts and able to provide the information I needed to meet the goals of my research. While it has been my experience that snowball sampling is an adequate segue into a community, criteria refinement is still needed to obtain information-rich data. For example, I have conducted studies with African American cancer survivors but found it necessary to refine my criteria to a specific African American cancer survivor. I needed to consider phase in the cancer journey, type treatment, time since treatment, etc. In my previous research, I have had to specify whether the best informants had a solid tumor cancer, late vs early-stage diagnosis, during the time of diagnosis, during chemotherapy treatment, or within one year of diagnosis. I specifically have found that the best information-rich data has come from those African Americans whose lives have been changed from their diagnosis; i.e., a change in appearance or loss of employment.

Saturation and Qualitative Research

Probably the more nebulous of all concepts associated with qualitative research methods is saturation. When this concept is used in proposals and manuscripts, I immediately question: Saturation of what? Saturation how? Saturation of information? Saturation of themes? Saturation of categories? Is it possible to determine saturation too early? How confident are you that you achieved saturation? This section discusses saturation as a determination of sample size; what appears to be standard practice, and why more rigor is needed in this area.

In the review of manuscripts and even in my own work, the term saturation is used loosely without detail. A frequently used statement is "Participants were interviewed or will be interviewed until the point of saturation" or "participants interviewed until the point of informational redundancy or theoretical saturation." These statements appear to satisfy some reviewers' criteria for the determination of sample size, while other reviewers will only accept that a sample size in qualitative research is adequate if a standard number reaches 20–30 as suggested by experts of qualitative methods (Creswell & Baez, 2021). Although there is no predetermined number at the outset of a study when saturation will be achieved, I have also found it difficult to justify a sample that is less than 30. It's like the reviewer is saying, "yea, I hear you say you achieved saturation, but I don't believe saturation is possible if the sample size is less than some magical number in my mind."

Data Saturation/Theoretical Saturation

Data saturation and informational redundancy in the determination of an adequate sample size are terms used interchangeably. However, the mere use of these terms does not inform the reader as to the specificities of information that is saturated. In the examples below, I describe ways in which I determined saturation.

Study Title: Types of Social Support among Elderly African American Cancer Patients.
Purpose/Objectives: To determine the types of social support elderly African Americans use to cope with the experience of cancer.
Research Approach: Qualitative study using a grounded theory approach.
Setting: Participant's homes in the Southeastern United States.

Participants: A purposive sample of 13 African American men (61–79 years) treated for prostate cancer and 15 African American women (42–87 years) treated for breast cancer. Participants selected according to key variables known to influence social support—age, gender, marital status, education, geographic region, and proximity to family.

Methodologic Approach: Open-ended and semi-structured interviews conducted with each participant N = 28). Interviews aimed at eliciting descriptions of the participants' experiences with social support during diagnosis, treatment, and post-treatment periods. Participants interviewed until informational redundancy was achieved. Constant comparison techniques are used to identify variations of social support both within cases and across cases.

Main Research Variable: The experience of social support among African Americans with cancer.

Findings: Participants used types of social support not currently emphasized in literature. The emotional support of "presence" was most frequently reported. Instrumental support included current conceptualizations but also offers of prayers, assistance to continue religious practices and assistance to maintain social roles. Informational support included what to expect, how to manage symptoms, help to interpret information, and validation of information received.

Conclusions: These findings suggest the need to reconceptualize social support for African Americans with cancer and to refine instruments to include these different manifestations of social support.

Nursing Implications: Researchers can use these findings in the design of culturally relevant questionnaires and interventions for this population. Clinicians can use knowledge of the types of social support valued among African American cancer patients to develop more appropriate strategies to promote healthy outcomes for this population.

In this research study, types of social support among African Americans with cancer, I was monitoring for saturation throughout data collection and data analysis. Recall, my overall goal was to construct a typology of social support that was culturally relevant for African American cancer survivors. I started the study with a conceptualization of social support that consisted of three components—emotional support, instrumental support, and informational support. Each subcategory of social support was related and comprised a larger conceptualization of social support.

Data collection and analysis were guided by this conceptualization of social support in addition to the integration of constant comparison and maximum sampling. Constant comparison was used to discern patterns and variations in the types of support both within and across cases while maximum variation was used to ensure a diverse sample. For example, I would explore the data for types of emotional, instrumental, and informational support as well as for sampling among a diverse population of African American cancer survivors. I would interview African American women who were well-educated about their experiences with social support, then once saturation was achieved among this group, I would explore the social support experiences among women with low levels of education; women who were married; never married, etc. Once I was saturated with the women with the variables known to influence the experience of social support,

I proceeded to interview men. Then in the same order, men who were highly educated, low levels of education, married vs. never married, etc. In this study, data saturation occurred regardless of how I structured the interview questions around the social support experience, the context within which social support was transacted among the subgroups of participants did not change.

In the previous example, theoretical sampling was used to understand properties of categories/subcategories of social support. Theoretical sampling could have also been useful to define the antecedents and consequences of the type of social support used. Time constraints, limited resources, and especially participant burden hindered this in-depth exploration and generation of a tentative theory of social support that could have included the context of the supportive interactions that occur among African American cancer survivors. In this next study to exploring context of social support interactions, informational redundancy was used to determine the adequacy of the sample size.

Data Saturation/Informational Redundancy

Data saturation and informational redundancy in the determination of an adequate sample size are terms used interchangeably. However, the mere use of these terms does not inform the reader as to the specificities of information that is saturated. In the example below, I describe ways in which I determined saturation through informational redundancy. No new information emerged during data collection in response to interview questions focused on events surrounding social support interactions.

Study Title: Perceptions of Support and Care Needs among Older African American Cancer Survivors.

Purpose/Objective: To explore the perceived support and care needs among older African American cancer survivors.

Design: Qualitative design using grounded theory techniques.

Sample: Focus groups with 22 older African American cancer survivors.

Methods: Purposeful sampling technique was used to identify participants from outpatient oncology clinics in the southeastern United States. In-depth interviews were conducted during treatment, post-treatment, and long-term follow-up care. Participants were interviewed until informational redundancy was achieved.

Findings: Support and care needs of these survivors were influenced by: (1) symptoms and treatment side effects; (2) perceptions of stigma and fears expressed among family and friends; (3) cultural beliefs about cancer; and (4) desires to lessen any burden or disruption to the lives of family and friends. Survivors discussed how these factors affected their social support experiences, how they navigated within and outside of their usual social networks to get their support and care needs met, and how their emotional well-being was affected.

Conclusions: The support from family, friends, and fellow church members is important to positive health outcomes among older African American cancer survivors. Yet, misconceptions, fears, and cultural beliefs about cancer negatively influence these traditional sources of support.

Implications for Nursing: Early identification of the factors that influence social support and care needs of this population can facilitate strategies to enhance positive outcomes and decrease health disparities among this population.

During data collection, support and care needs of these African Americans emerged: (1) symptoms and treatment side effects; (2) perceptions of stigma and fears expressed among family and friends; (3) cultural beliefs about cancer; and (4) desires to lessen any burden or disruption to the lives of family and friends. To arrive at informational redundancy, I interviewed participants about these topics until the point that no new information emerged. Initial interviews were unstructured and began with a general question that asked: "Tell me how cancer has affected your life." Other general questions that pursued were "Did relationships with family and friends change?" "What were your experiences with negative beliefs, attitudes, and behaviors toward you after the cancer diagnosis?" Questions were designed to promote open discussions of support and care needs affected by the cancer experience from the survivors' perspective and reflected the interviewer's prior sensitization to concepts in health-related and historical literature on social support and social networks. As the interviews progressed, questions became more directed and pursued analytic lines that emerged in previous interviews. Probing questions were asked throughout the interviews to encourage participants to talk about events important to their cancer experiences to the point where no new information emerged in each category or theme that emerged during data collection and analysis.

Conclusion

This chapter focused on sampling strategies useful in qualitative research among an underserved population of African American cancer survivors. I described ways in which I used types of purposive sampling (convenient, criterion, maximum variation, theoretical, snowball). As you have seen, in the conduct of research among underserved communities, sampling strategies were not used in isolation. Convenient sampling may be needed to gain entry into the community and to determine the appropriate purposeful sample. Even when the criterion for the sample has been identified, the addition of maximum variation may be necessary for a diverse population.

In this chapter, I also included a discussion on issues with saturation. Researchers habitually state in manuscripts that the sample size was determined by saturation. However, little description follows about the process for saturation, whether it was informational redundancy or theoretical saturation, and how saturation was achieved. Given that reviewers tend to be quantitatively oriented in their approach to science, they may have expectations that a specific number of participants are necessary to achieve saturation.

In Chapter 6, the conversation continues with a focus on the interview with particular considerations for privacy, research burden, constructing interview questions, and probing questions. In Chapter 7, I discuss my experience with focus groups vs. the semi-structured interview. I also continue the discussion of interviewing with examples to achieve saturation.

References

Broman, C. L. (1991). "Gender, work-family roles, and psychological well-being of blacks." *J Marriage Fam* **53**: 509–520.

Brown, D. R., and L. E., Gary (1985). "Social support network differentials among married and nonmarried black females." *Psychol Women Q* **9**: 229–241.

Brown, D. R. and L. E. Gary (1987). "Stressful life events, social support networks, and the physical and mental health of urban black adults." *J Human Stress* **13**(4): 165–174.

Chatters, L. M., R. J. Taylor and R. Jayakody (1994). "Fictive kinship relations in black extended families." *J Comp Fam Stud* **25**(3): 297–312.
Creswell, J. W. and J. C. Baez (2021). *30 Essential Skills for the Qualitative Researcher*. Thousand Oaks, CA, Sage Publishing.
Dressler, W. W. (1985). "Extended family relationships, social support, and mental health in a Southern Black community." *Psychosom Med* **53**: 608–620.
Hamilton, J. B., C. E. Moore, B. D. Powe, M. Agarwal and P. Martin (2010). "Perceptions of support among older African American cancer survivors." *Oncol Nurs Forum* **37**(4): 484–493.
Hatch, L. R. (1991). "Informal support patterns of older African-American and white women." *Res Aging* **13**(2): 144–170.
Jayakody, R., L. Chatters and R. J. Taylor (1993). Family support to single and married African American mothers: The provision of financial, emotional, and child care assistance." *J Marriage Fam* **55**: 261–276.
Jones, J. (1995). *Labor of Love, Labor of Sorrow*. New York, Vintage Books.
Kahn, R. L. and T. C. Antonucci (1980). Convoys Over the Life Course: Attachment, Roles, and Social Support. *Life-Span Development and Behavior*. P. B. Baltes and O. G. Grim. New York, Academic Press. **3**: 253–286.
Lincoln, C. E. (1974). *The Black Church Since Frazier*. New York, Schocken Books.
Mathews, H. F., D. R. Lannin and J. P. Mitchell (1994). "Coming to terms with advanced breast cancer: Black women's narratives from Eastern North Carolina." *Soc Sci Med* **38**(6): 789–800.
Maxwell, J. A. (2013). *Qualitative Research Design: An Interactive Approach*. Thousand Oaks, CA, Sage Publications, Inc.
Merriam, S. B. and E. J. Tisdell (2016). *Qualitative Research: A Guide to Design and Implementation*. San Francisco, CA, Jossey-Bass.
Neighbors, H. W. and C. S. Howard (1987). "Sex differences in professional help seeking among adult black Americans." *Am J Community Psychol* **15**(4): 403–417.
Neighbors, H. W. and J. S. Jackson (1984). "The use of informal and formal help: Four patterns of illness behavior in the black community." *Am J Community Psychol* **12**(6): 629–644.
Powdermaker, H. (1937/1993). *After Freedom: A Cultural Study in the Deep South*. Madison, WS, University of Wisconsin Press.
Primomo, J., B. C. Yates and N. F. Woods (1990). "Social support for women during chronic illness: The relationship among sources and types to adjustment." *Res Nurs Health* **13**: 153–161.
Strauss, A. and J. Corbin (1998). *Basics of Qualitative Research*. Thousand Oaks, CA, Sage Publications.
Strauss, A. L. (1999). *Qualitative Analysis for Social Scientists*. Cambridge, UK, Cambridge University Press.
Taylor, R. J., C. B. Hardison and L. M. Chatters (1996). Kin and nonkin as sources of informal assistance. *Mental Health in Black America*. H. W. Neighbors and J. S. Jackson (Eds.). Newbury Park, CA: Sage: 130–145.
Walls, C. T. (1992). "The role of church and family support in the lives of older African-Americans." *Generations* (Summer): 33–36.

6 The Art and Science of Data Collection for SDOH in Community Engaged Research (Part 1)

As a PhD student, I remember enrolling in the introductory qualitative methods course and reading the content on data collection in the assigned texts. I recall still asking my mentors at the time, "what questions do I ask"? I was a nurse and should have been comfortable talking to patients, but I was a MICU nurse and the majority of our patients were intubated and couldn't talk. What I did have was a background where I was raised in a small close community of elders. I was raised by my grandmother who was probably the greatest storyteller ever, plus I loved listening to folk tell their stories. However, prior to my first interview, I was extremely nervous. In Chapters 6 and 7, I will share those early experiences to enable you to have a less stressful experience and obtain the best story(s) for your research project. In Chapter 6 (Part 1 of Data Collection), I begin the conversation on data collection with topics related to preparation for the interview. In Chapter 7 (Part 2 of Data Collection), I continue the conversation on data collection to discuss topics related to the actual interview.

This chapter contains information related to preparation for data collection:

- The setting
- Interviewer as instrument
- Considerations for respect during interviews
- Culturally appropriate interview questions
- Number of interview questions

The Setting

The majority of the content in this chapter focuses on the participant and the interview. However, a major factor in data collection not frequently talked about is where the data will be collected. Oftentimes, we broadly state for the IRB application that data will be collected at a facility or the home, or other location convenient for the participant. In this section, I would like to offer some of my experiences with data collection in various settings. Specifically, I will discuss those settings and the pros and cons of data in those settings (homes, churches, clinics, academic settings, telephone, and video conferencing. Of all the places or settings that I have conducted interviews for my qualitative research projects, the participant's home is my preference.

Participant home. I find that the participant home is the setting that places the participant in a familiar environment which is likely the most comfortable for them to share their experience. Older participants may not be as mobile and prefer their home. I have also found that participants in remote rural areas love the visit, so be prepared to "sit a spell."

DOI: 10.4324/9781003598916-6

However, there are pros and cons when the participant's home is the setting. Data collection in the participant's home can be a burden to both interviewer and interviewee. The interviewer has to have the flexibility in their schedule to travel. Traveling can also be time-intensive and risky. I have been fortunate in that the homes I traveled to were in physically safe environments, and I was never in an unsafe environment. Concerns with traveling include whether the home is in a safe location, whether the car I am driving might break down, and whether I have all the equipment needed since I am not able to quickly return to the office to retrieve needed equipment. I have always been careful to schedule interviews so that I am not on the road after dark, and I always inform members of my team where I am traveling. At one time, I was able to take my son with me when traveling to remote rural areas to conduct interviews. He was helpful with directions and reading road signs, so I didn't get lost. He also assisted in carrying equipment from the car into the house, collecting signed informed consent forms, and distributing gift cards. As previously stated, travel to participant homes is time-intensive, and I have never been able to do more than two in-person interviews in any given day because of the time it takes to drive from one home to the next. Finally, when conducting interviews in participant homes, be aware of cultural values and expectations for behavior so as not the offend the host. Offer to take shoes off at the door, use greetings that are appropriate, and stay only as long as you agreed to. There have been times when participants wanted to show me pictures or introduce me to family members. Try to be brief with preinterview conversations, so you get the information you came for. You may think it is okay to stay longer since they were talking but after you leave, they will remember that your visit was longer than expected and kept them from doing their chores. They may remember this and not invite you (or any other researcher) to return. A final word about food. For some communities, it is a welcoming gesture to offer food and drink to visitors. Use your judgment when accepting food or drink. I generally will accept something to drink and pass on any food (for health reasons). Another option is to take food (cookies, fruit) or drink as a friendly gesture to the participant. Whatever you do, when in a participant's home, be respectful.

Participant church. I have occasionally interviewed clergy in their church office and participants in a private church classroom. This is a convenient setting since you can conduct the interview right before or immediately after a planned activity. The interview with clergy has worked well since they have access to the church office at any time and can schedule the interview when the church is quiet. Conducting the interview before or after a church activity, even in a private classroom, is not as good. It is difficult to control noise from nearby rooms, and the interview has often felt rushed since access to the church building is restricted. While not my preference, I was able to interview some participants that I otherwise would not have had access to.

Clinic setting. Conducting the participant interview in the clinic setting is probably on the same level as that in the private church classroom. I have used consulting rooms, empty exam rooms, and even unused waiting rooms. These rooms worked well in that they were convenient for the participant, and I could schedule the interview on an infusion day, laboratory draw day, or follow-up clinic day. These visits should be scheduled prior to the clinic appointment since participants are frequently tired after the clinic visit or may have a ride waiting. Interviews in unused waiting rooms worked best, but you always risk the chance that the room will be needed. Always have a plan B for if this happens. Never, ever, schedule an interview in the clinic cafeteria. It is noisy, you can't hear them, and they can't hear you. I have even tried the local coffee shop. Same issues.

Academic setting. Conducting the participant interview in a private room in your school or department is without question, extremely convenient to the interviewer. However, for the interviewee make sure you have provided clear directions for travel, for parking, and access to the building. For parking, provide passes or cash disbursement to lessen the burden of travel to the interviewee. If the interview is close to meal time, providing food and drink is a nice gesture.

Telephone. For older African Americans, communicating via telephone is second to face-to-face, and my preference when face-to-face is not possible. With telephone communications, the conversation is focused soley on verbal expressions. There is no travel time for the interviewee, no parking, and it is less likely that there will be interruptions from others. However, there is still the concern that the telephone interview is scheduled for a time when both interviewer and interviewee are quietly sitting someplace and not driving or needing to move locations during the interview. I recall having a scheduled interview (I was the interviewee), and the interviewer was driving. I could hear the noise in the car and her voice going in and out. I paused and asked if she was driving. She was. Clearly, my interview was not important to her. I ended the interview and asked her to call me back when the time was more convenient for her.

Video conferencing. Conducting the face-to-face interview via video conferencing format can be convenient for both interviewer and interviewee and can be cost-effective, not requiring the cost of travel. Technology, however, can be unreliable and erratic, and delays in the signal can be extremely distracting and disruptive to the flow of conversation. While interviewing via video conferencing uses the latest in technology, this form of communication is limited to interviewees with wi-fi access and the knowledge to navigate this technology. Older adults in remote rural areas or anyone not accustomed to the world of technology might be excluded from research requiring this form of technology. Excluding these populations would suppress their voices in future research that seeks to develop or adapt measures and interventions.

Interviewer as Instrument

In the quantitative research project, the data collector approaches the research subject with a well-crafted series of questions that have been evaluated for reliability and validity and tested for language and cultural relevance among the target population. Data collectors are trained to be consistent in asking the questions, to ensure there is no missing data. For consistency in data collection, there are to be no changes in the language of the questions and no changes in the order of the questions during data collection. Data collection during a quantitative study is structured, consisting of closed-ended questions with the ability to obtain numerical data to test hypotheses, identify patterns, and ultimately generalize findings to a larger population (Carminati, 2018; Tabachnick & Fidell, 2018). Completed questionnaires from large numbers of subjects are necessary to achieve power for statistical significance. The larger the numbers of questionnaires completed (sample size), the greater the inference of reliability and generalizability of findings (Carminati, 2018; Tabachnick & Fidell, 2018).

Recall the goal of qualitative research is to derive an understanding, meanings, or experiences of some phenomenon. Data collected can be through non-numerical data, stories, documents, diaries, or even observations. As such, data collection with qualitative methods doesn't follow the same rules as in quantitative methods. Data collection during a qualitative study is minimally structured, consisting of open-ended or semi-structured questions to generate tentative theory, refine conceptualizations, and understand unique illness experiences. The ultimate goal of a qualitative project is to collect information-rich data from an in-depth exploration with small number of participants who are experts on a phenomenon; to ultimately generate knowledge that can be transferred or applied to other situations or settings, or to develop or adapt measures or interventions. Obtaining information-rich data in a project using qualitative methods is largely dependent on the skill of the instrument, which in qualitative research is the interviewer. In my opinion, there are three critical skills for the qualitative data collector: (1) be a good listener; (2) be comfortable with silence; and 3) be calm during emotional reactions.

Be a good listener. When planning for the interview and responding to IRB requirements, qualitative researchers compile a list of questions to be asked during the interview. When my input is requested, I always respond with the question "if you go into the interview with 20 questions for a 60-minute interview, when will the participant have time to talk about topics important to them?" The approach of having a long list of questions prior to the interview assumes that the researcher already knows the questions they want answered, leaving no time for participants to share experiences that are unanticipated or an unexpected direction. Qualitative data collectors skilled at listening are able to start the interview with a few questions, and depending on the interview, follow the flow of the interview, probing as needed to capture the experience.

Be comfortable with silence. Early in my career, I was very uncomfortable when the interviewee would pause during the interview. I thought that I needed to quickly ask another question from my list to keep the conversation going. As I gained experience and became more comfortable during interviews, I wasn't nervous with pauses. These pauses allowed participants to gather their thoughts and continue the interview with topics important to them. Oftentimes, these conversations led to previously unexplored experiences that changed the direction of my program of research.

Be calm during emotional reactions. As previously mentioned, I was a bedside nurse before I became a scientist. As a nurse, you are trained to comfort the patient, to alleviate suffering, to communicate hope during stressful life situations. This instinct to care for the patient often led to my wanting to give advice during the interview or change the topic when patients became emotionally upset. I recall during a one-on-one interview, a participant teared up during the response to one of my research questions. I asked if she wanted to stop the interview or talk about something else. To my surprise, she said no, that I was the only person she had to talk to about the topic. We continued the interview, and as a result, I learned about an experience that enriched my research.

Considerations for Respect During Interviews

In Chapter 2, I discuss strategies for being respectful when conducting research in the community. These strategies also apply during the conduct of the interview in qualitative research.

Respect for the interviewee's home or other personal space. During the conduct of qualitative research, scientists may collect data in the private spaces of participant homes or spaces in faith-based institutions. When entering these spaces, it is critical to be respectful. This respect is inclusive of participant's traditions, values, and history. Respect shown to participants is important even if the qualitative research is conducted in health care settings or other public spaces.

Probably the most important display of respect is in the way individuals are addressed during initial interactions. It is important to be knowledgeable of the cultural background of participants and address them appropriately during interactions. Prior to the interview, I am always careful to know an individual's age, educational degree, and role occupied in the home, as leaders in community organizations, or in faith-based institutions. The first rule during interactions is that I never address an older person by their first name. *Never*. Do not ask the individual if it is okay, it is not. In remote rural communities where I was raised, older persons were addressed as Mr. or Mrs., Uncle [first name] or Aunt [first name], or Cousin [first name]. Older individuals who were close like family members were addressed as Mr. or Miss followed by the first name. Extended older family members were addressed as Aunt or Uncle followed by their first name. Everyone else is addressed as Mr. or Mrs. and their last name. For individuals in faith-based institutions, it is important to understand titles and address individuals appropriately. For example, you may need to address faith-based leaders appropriately as Bishop, Elder, Pastor, or Reverend and Deacon. Some clergy may have earned doctorates in ministry and therefore should be addressed as Dr. followed by their last names. These individuals have worked hard to earn these titles and desire to be appropriately addressed as such.

Respect for traditions and social norms. These traditions and social norms may include how individuals celebrate religious traditions, holidays, birthdays, or funerals. Among the communities where I have conducted research, Sundays are generally designated days for religious services; Thanksgiving, Christmas, Easter, and the Fourth of July are times of family gatherings and celebrations in African American communities. When recruitment and data collection are scheduled during these dates, I always pause recruiting efforts and data collection to later dates if possible.

Considerations for mealtimes. There have been a few times when I scheduled focus groups during the lunch or dinner hour. For these occasions, I always have food, snacks, fruit, and beverages available for participants. However, when traveling to participant's homes, I try to avoid scheduling interviews at high noon or the 5 or 6 pm dinner hour. In addition to not wanting to disrupt mealtimes, I want to avoid making participants feel obligated to feed me. I did not follow this advice when I first started scheduling interviews. Not sure if this is still customary, but in previous years in rural communities, it was customary to offer food and drink to visitors. Not wanting to be offensive, I would politely refuse food but always accept something to drink.

Keeping promises. The interviewer should clearly articulate the purpose of the study in a language familiar to the participant. Participants should be informed of the questions they will be asked, how interviews will be conducted, and most importantly, who will see their information and how that information will be used.

Considerations for participant time and incentives. Show up as promised, stay only as long as promised, and distribute incentives as promised. Showing up as promised is simply being on time to appointments. If you need to cancel, arrange for someone else to go in your place. They may have rearranged their day to accommodate your visit, and they should be your priority. When traveling in remote rural areas on roads I am not familiar with or even when I find myself stuck in traffic or behind a slow-driving car on a two-lane country road, I pull over and phone ahead to let the participant know that I will be late and why. I have been late to more than one appointment because I made a wrong turn (Google Maps was confused). When I arrived, the participant was sitting outside in a lawn chair waiting for me. Oftentimes, for older participants in the country, you may be their only visitor for the day, and they will be waiting for you to show up.

Do not exceed the time you told them to conduct the interview. If the interview is taking longer than expected, remember you are changing your contract with them. Any changes to what you told them about the interview need to be renegotiated. You need to get their permission to stay longer than planned. While it may appear that participants are enjoying the interview and just now opening up about their experiences, they will remember that you stayed longer than you said and kept them from other activities they had planned for the day. Better to pause and get permission to stay longer, or even better arrange for a second follow-up interview. I have done these follow-up interviews by phone, which has worked well.

A final word about the distribution of incentives. Cash (not checks) may be best if at all possible. The distribution of incentives in the form of gift cards is less burdensome than cash. However, for gift cards to be usable, the researcher needs some knowledge of the local environment and purchase cards that can be easily used. Lastly, I have always distributed any incentive prior to the start of the interview. That is, when asking participants to sign the consent form, I go ahead and have them sign for the incentive so that the remainder of our time is focused on the interview. My rationale for distributing incentives prior to the interview is that they are not distracted during the interview, wondering whether you are really going to give them what you have promised.

Although not a promise, if possible, I feel that it is important to let the participant see how their stories were used and to also give them access to their stories for their own uses. For example, I have given participants copies of papers published in academic journals that they would otherwise not have access to. I have also presented findings to educational programs and health fairs sponsored by support groups of which participants were members.

Culturally Sensitive and Appropriate Interview Questions

In this section, I describe culturally sensitive (an awareness) and culturally appropriate (a responsiveness) to interview questions. My approach to this topic is through my lens as an African American, of Baptist and AME affiliations, rural background, highly educated, and Professor at a predominantly white research institution. When I approach interviewees, I am careful to remember to bracket my beliefs and biases so as not to impose them on the interviewee and hinder the expression of their perspectives. Asking questions that are sensitive to the interviewee and not offensive requires knowledge of the interviewees culture and even historical background. Even if the interviewer is of a similar culture and historical background, care is needed to refrain from assumptions around beliefs, jargon, or other language that may illicit negative emotions. Considerations in the conduct of research with African Americans are the heterogeneity among the population, power dynamics between interviewer and interviewee, and the potential for social responsibility bias.

Specifically, during the conduct of research with African American populations, I have been reminded that although I grew up in the communities where I was raised, in some ways I am similar but also different. Revealing these similarities and differences during the interview could influence the data I am able to obtain. For example, I grew up in the Baptist Church among Evangelicals but no longer believe everything I was taught in my early years. I am reminded that I have access to financial and educational resources that a majority of my interviewees do not have. This lack of financial and educational resources has limited the African American population's ability to access higher education. Interviewers need to be careful that interviewees are not made to feel "less than" during interactions. A final reminder is that as a heterogeneous population, individual African Americans may not possess any of the beliefs or values typically ascribed to the dominant African American culture.

Rather than provide a list of example interview questions, I would suggest a list of considerations for interview questions. These considerations should include:

1 *Whether the language or wording of questions is familiar or understood.*

  During my dissertation, my research question was to understand the social support experiences of African American cancer survivors? I knew from my experiences with the population that social support was not a frequently used language to describe the helping that occurred during illness situations. Instead of the academic language of asking "Tell me about your social support?," I used the familiar language of "Tell me what helped you?" I was also mindful that my long-term goal with this research was to develop a culturally sensitive measure of social support, and wanted to capture the language (expression of words) used among this population to capture the support actually used when constructing items for the new questionnaire.

2 *Whether the questions are forcing participants to respond according to assumptions about the larger population, ignoring the heterogeneity or subcultures that exist.*

  Probably the better example for this consideration is the strong religious culture that exists among African Americans. This cultural influence can lead the interviewer to assume that all African Americans are religious and believe in God. Similarly, the African American interviewee may not feel comfortable answering questions about religion or spirituality when they don't attend church regularly or even believe that God exists.

3 *Whether the questions will cause emotional distress.*

  It is impossible to know at the outset, exactly which questions may trigger anger, sadness, or anxieties. I think it is safe to assume that questions about loss, separation, fear, isolation, grief that are associated with SDOH topics are likely to cause some emotional distress. I suggest that these questions be asked as late as possible in the interview. Be prepared to pause or stop the interview if needed and have a referral should participants continue to be distressed at the end of the interview.

4 *Whether the questions will make participants appear or feel weak.*

  For the older African American especially, a history of oppression and racism is likely to have influenced an internalized value of needing to be strong even in adverse situations. Older African Americans who have integrated this value into their self-concept may reject thoughts or behaviors that make them appear or feel weak. This is especially apparent during illness when the older African American who has been socialized to be strong, to have faith in God, and to not be a burden on others. During interview questions, I am mindful of my achievements as a well-educated African American woman to structure questions around education and income in a way that does not cause anyone that I interview to feel inferior or less than.

  When asking cancer patients questions about *social support,* I am aware of a prevailing view of cancer as a death sentence that persists in spite of the advances made in cancer treatment. The lack of positive cancer survivorship stories that circulate among African American communities has caused families, friends, coworkers, and fellow church congregants to be fearful of a cancer diagnosis. Supportive relationships may be lacking, and attempts to provide support may be inappropriate. Additionally, African Americans may live in geographical locations with little or no access to facilities that offer cancer screening. As a result, African Americans encountered in the community and recruited into our research may have later staged cancer diagnoses that should have been prevented. Interview questions should be structured to consider that there are SDOH influences on the individual cancer experience. Care should be taken not to communicate through the interview question that the participant is somehow to be blamed for their situation.

When the topic is *education*, I am aware that very few older African Americans who grew up during segregation attended college. In rural areas, older African Americans in my previous studies did not have access to high school, and their educational attainment was likely limited to what was available in their communities. When asking about education, I will structure the interview question to ask "How far were you able to go in school?" rather than asking "what is your highest level of education achieved?" Achieved has a connotation of personal responsibility when in fact participants from rural segregated parts of the country by law may have not been allowed to achieve their highest potential. Asking in this way lets the participant know that I am aware of the educational limitations placed on African Americans during their generation. Even when the interviewer is younger, only 26% of African Americans graduated with a bachelor's degree or higher in 2023.

Income is another sensitive topic for African Americans. It is well-known that African Americans have lower income levels when compared to their white counterparts. This disparity is attributed to the lower levels of education described previously, racism in the workplace, a lack of generational wealth, and overall financial hardships. In fact, the income levels for the older African American generally fall in the poverty range. Important to remember is that low levels of income may indicate a low purchasing power but not necessarily low intellect, as many older African Americans continued to informally educate themselves through community institutions or through adult children who did have access to higher educational institutions. During the interview, I am sensitive to this cultural and historical influence on income levels and only collect this information if it is critical to the research question. Even then, I will ask participants for an income range, never an exact number.

Number of Interview Questions

I have briefly discussed the number of interview questions appropriate for any given qualitative research study. Less is more. It is not unusual for the novice qualitative researcher to submit 15–20 interview questions for their project. An increased number of interview questions suggests that the interviewer already knows the specific information desired and no more. Fewer questions permit probing, gaining an in-depth exploration of the phenomenon of interest, and ultimately obtaining information-rich data for analysis. I typically submit to IRB 1–2 open-ended interview questions with examples of probing questions. A commitment to fewer interview questions serves two purposes: (1) It allows me to capture the story that is important to the participant and (2) It keeps me from having to do repeated modifications to IRB for permission to change interview questions.

Example 1 Interview Questions Submitted to IRB

The Development of a Spiritual Support Intervention for Older African Americans Encountering Stressful Life Events

During the interviews, the interviewer will obtain demographic information, and participants will be asked to talk about whether and how they use a religious song to help them with a stressful event such as a serious chronic or life-threatening illness. The interviews will consist of three open-ended questions:

1. *Can you recall a time in your life that was particularly stressful for you? Describe the illness and why it was stressful.*
2. *Tell me about a religious song that helped you during that time, and*
3. *Tell me how that song helped you during that time.*

Follow-up/probing questions include:

1. *Can you recall how you were feeling when you used that song? and*
2. *Tell me why you used that particular song?*

Conclusion

This chapter covers my experiences with the aspect of data collection that relates to preparation for the interview during research focused on SDOH using qualitative methods. I began with issues related to the setting and closed with a discussion on issues related to the development of culturally sensitive interview questions and decisions related to the appropriate number of interview questions prior to the interview. The next chapter concludes the discussion on data collection with a focus on the conduct of the actual interview. Specifically, I discuss types of interviews I have used in my research, when and how to conduct follow-up interviews, and the collection and recording of observation data during the interview.

References

Carminati, L. (2018). "Generalizability in qualitative research: A tale of two traditions." *Qual Health Res* **28**(13): 2094–2101.

Tabachnick, B. G. and L. S. Fidell. (2018). *Using Multivariate Statistics*. New York, Harpercollins College Publishers.

7 The Art and Science of Data Collection for SDOH in Community Engaged Research (Part 2)

In this chapter (Part 2 of Data Collection), I continue the conversation on data collection to discuss the actual interview on SDOH topics using qualitative research methods. Specifically, the topics in this chapter include:

- Focus group vs one-on-one interview
- Structure of interview questions (structured, unstructured, semi-structured)
- Conducting follow-up interviews
- Closing the interview
- A note on taking notes

Focus Group vs One-on-One Interview

In this section, I describe my experiences with focus groups and one-on-one interviews to understand the social support experiences of African American cancer survivors. The reader is referred to qualitative texts for content on the purposes and elements of each of these types of data collection.

Focus Group Interview

The focus group interview is the preferred type of data collection when the purpose of the research is to collect data from a group or groups of participants (Merriam & Tisdel, 2016; Morgan, 2019). The focus group is generally designed to capture data from participants talking to each other to gain their perspectives on a wide range of topics. In comparison to the one-on-one interview, the focus group is usually led by a moderator and interviewer, with the moderator guiding the discussion and managing group dynamics. As a form of data collection, focus groups can be a cost-effective method of reaching larger numbers of participants in a shorter period of time. The group interview is also believed to be empowering since this type of data collection allows participants to share their experiences with others and feel less isolated with their experiences during an interview. However, the focus group is likely not the best approach for the collection of sensitive data or topics of a private nature, although this view is controversial.

Recruitment for focus groups is similar to the one-on-one interview with the exception that each group works best if they contain between 4 and 6 participants. However, these smaller groups (each group is a unit) may offer less diversity than the project with one-on-one interviews. They may offer less time for discussion, and less opportunity for probing in unanticipated directions. Moreover, the group format that encourages agreement

DOI: 10.4324/9781003598916-7

and disagreement, may silence those participants who may feel shamed by their story by overly vocal participants. I have found while focus groups are an efficient method of data collection for the researcher, participation in a focus group is time-consuming for the participant. Time includes that for travel to a site that is convenient for the focus group, eating if refreshments are served, moderator instructions to the group, and the group interview, which can take 1.5–2 hours. In contrast, data collection for the one-on-one interview can take 45–60 minutes total.

In the sections below are examples of interview guides for a focus group of patients and family members. The second example is a transcript to illustrate the wording of an actual focus group of two African American cancer survivors. The purpose of the focus group interview was to learn more about the experience of cancer and perceptions of needed social support to develop a social support intervention.

Example 2 Focus Group Interview Guide (Cancer Patient)

1 What effect has cancer had on your quality of life?
By "quality of life" we mean your physical, psychological, and social health.
2 What symptoms/complications have you experienced that are troubling to you?
3 When you think about all the things that you have to manage related to this illness, what areas do you feel the most confident about?
4 If you were to develop an ideal or special program to help people live with cancer, what would you like to see in the program? What would you include to help your primary caregiver?

Example 3 Focus Group Interview Guide (Primary Caregiver)

5 What effect has cancer had on you? On your quality of life?
By "quality of life" we mean your physical, psychological, and social health.
6 What symptoms/complications have you seen experienced by the cancer patient that are troubling to you?
7 When you think about all the things the patient has to manage related to this illness, what areas do you feel the most confident about being able to help with?
8 If you were to develop an ideal or special program to help people live with cancer, what would you like to see in the program? What would you include to help other caregivers?

The example below is a partial transcript of a focus group with two African American men diagnosed with cancer. Although four men were invited to the focus group, only two actually showed up due to family emergencies. I was able to conduct one-on-one interviews with the two men not able to participate in the focus group.

Notice in the focus group how I began the conversation and ensured both participants understood the purpose of the study using a language that I believed comfortable for them. In spite of this being the first time these two individuals had met, the flow of the conversation was respectful and neither individuals' responses were influenced by the others. During the interview, I followed the topics that emerged during the questioning; seeking clarification from each participant. The interview was informative and with probing, I was able to learn about each individual's source of social support and the types of social support derived from that source.

Example 4 Partial Transcript of Focus Group Interview

Interviewer:	Okay. So I got about five questions and just … I want you … this to be done … okay, now … okay so the first question is … if you could talk to me a little bit about … and we can go all the way back as far as you can remember when you were diagnosed … and talk to me a little bit about, um, the support that you got from family and friends. Who were some of the key players, um, and who you talk to … just about, you know, the relationship with people around you, um, the support they gave you. What was good – what was not good? What you, um, what you received and what you would have liked to have received more of from people around you that could have been, you know … um, talk about, you know, support from your wife, family and friends, relatives, church, work … well you retired, so that wouldn't … but church, your community, and I know some of it was positive and just pos … the good and the bad … positive and negative.
1st Man:	Okay.
Interviewer:	Hold on. Okay, so I got about five questions to ask. Okay. And the first questions is, talk to me about the people that helped you when you got your diagnosis of cancer.
1st Man	Yeah.
2nd Man:	Yeah.
1st Man:	Um-hmm.
Interviewer:	… what, what kinds of things that you go from people … what kind of help did you get that was good and what was not so good? Okay?
1st Man:	With all the information I received, um, while making these appointments, proved therapeutic … very, very, very therapeutic. And it also gave me hope … a lot of faith in myself.
Interviewer:	Um-hmm.
1st Man:	And I was also enlightened about some of the dangers, uh, I would have had, had I not gone … undergone the treatment.
Interviewer:	Okay. Who were some of the people that helped you?
1st Man:	"G". "G" helped me a lot, and …
Interviewer:	"G", the young man here?
1st Man:	Yes, the one that, uh, is a counselor. Um, he gave me a lot of hope.
Interviewer:	"G" did?
1st Man	Yes, "G" did. And then I was treated more that good by the nurses…
Interviewer:	Um-hmm.
1st Man:	… and staff.
Interviewer:	Um-hmm.

1st Man:	I found them to be more than courteous, understanding, and that just about wraps it up.
Interviewer:	What about anybody in your family? Do you have any family?
1st Man:	Yes, I have family. Um, I discussed it with my family and, and they, they didn't feel fearful in any way. Uh, they always by my side. I can always depend on them. When I'm in need of anything.
Interviewer:	Um-hmm.
1st Man:	So I have faith. My faith is strong too. I have … I pray …
Interviewer:	Um-hmm.
1st Man:	… meditate, um, every day. And I find all that supporting.
Interviewer:	Okay. You wanna talk some here now?
2nd Man:	Why certainly…listening to him, my case is a little different. I guess, um, but um … when I first found out from the … my internal medicine doctor … recommended the, the test. And of course, the, uh, neurologist did the test and uh, told me the results. He said, he said that I would … told me all my options and uh, he, he was a surgeon. And of course, uh, I went to a radiologist. He also recommended I talk to all the people with that type, it's prostate cancer. And um, they were all … told me what to expect, what, you know, told me everything I needed to know. And uh, I made this, this decision. I made the decision of which type of uh, treatment to take. And uh, discussed it with my wife, who was with me during the, during the uh, each of the meetings. And uh, initially, uh … obviously, it was very uh, it was real hard when you find out that you … you do have cancer.
Interviewer:	Um-hmm.
2nd Man:	It was for me, of course, uh, my family was supportive. The treatment was, was successful so far so I feel good about that.
Interviewer:	Will you tell me … talk … tell me some about what it was like, um, telling people, um, over the course, about … maybe … did you have to ever ask for any kind of help or support from family?
2nd Man:	No, um, I, actually I only told my wife. And of course I, uh, made the decision to tell my son. And uh, he was uh 14 at the time. Um, and, uh, of course, I think the word got out from them to the other relatives. Then they all, you know, called, and, and expressed whatever help I needed.
Interviewer:	Um-hmm.
2nd Man:	But that's pretty … it was very small group of people that were … that know.
Interviewer:	Um-hmm.
2nd Man:	Um, the support was there from them, but, uh, everything was … everything was good. There was no bad experiences.
Interviewer:	Okay. What about, um, were you involved with a church?
2nd Man:	I, I regularly attend church. And it's … that I would say helped me get through everything.
Interviewer:	The church?

2nd Man: Emotionally, yes.

Interviewer: Okay.

2nd Man: But as far as actively, uh, anyone at church that knew … very few knew.

Interviewer: Why was that?

2nd Man: I just … I'm a very private, private person. So I didn't … I was dealing with it. Treatments were going well.

Interviewer: Um-hmm.

2nd Man: And uh, I'm just hoping and looking towards, you know, positive, you know. But I don't, don't speak too much about it to anyone other than the family.

Interviewer: What about the minister? Was he involved?

2nd Man: I, I, I told one of the assistant pastors. And uh, you know, she said we'll pray for you. And uh, but I wasn't, you know, in my case, it wasn't, you know, in my case, it wasn't, um, everything was going so well that it's more, you know, praying your recovery continues …

Interviewer: Okay.

2nd Man: … as oppose to; you know

Interviewer: Okay. Um, let me ask you this. I'm a skip it and I may come back. One of the things, "Mr. S" … one of the things that some other men have said is that they worried about when they got, um, treatment and maybe some of them lost weight, they worried about how they looked, around other people. Was that ever an issue or problem for you, losing weight and …

2nd Mind No.

Interviewer: … how you might look?

2nd Man: No … I … never crossed my mind.

Interviewer: Okay.

2nd Man: Not mine.

Interviewer: Okay. Go to the next question. This is the next one. Um, a lot of times, you know, you, "Mr. S", you talked about your faith and praying …

1st Man: Yeah.

Interviewer: Okay. Did you every have people to, um, come and pray with you? Or people tell you they gonna pray for you?

1st Man: Yes.

Interviewer: Okay. The other thing is … this is really my question. I know that they rely heavily on their faith and they pray a lot. Um, hmm, but were there ever times that you wanted to talk about issues related to spirituality. And maybe sometimes you worried in spite of, say having a strong faith. Should I reword that?

Both Men Yes.

Interviewer: Okay. I know that over the years, I've been told that people relied heavily on their spiritually. They turned it over to God. Or they prayed to God and they have faith that God will bring them through. But were there ever times … see, my, my thoughts are that. And I've talked to other people. But still, sometimes people try to find meaning in that experience – for example, they may have said, well, why did this happen to me? And they look to scriptures to try to figure out why this happen to me. Did you ever have a need to talk to anybody about those kinds of issues? Okay?

2nd Man: Not, not, not me.

Interviewer: Okay. What about you "Mr. S"?

1st Man: Well, I know when I was in the service, uh, I had to have a spinal shot … spinal tap.

Interviewer: Um-hmm.

1st Man: And before the doctor, uh, administered the, the needle in my spine, he said for me not to move, that it might paralyze you …

Interviewer: Um-hmm.

1st Man: … and, well, I had … that was the greatest fear I ever had in my life, and um …

Interviewer: More so than even the cancer?

1st Man: Yes and, and I, I still rely on my prayer.

Interviewer: Um-hmm.

1st Man: My faith in God.

Interviewer: Um-hmm.

1st Man: I came to death on two occasions and God has brought me through. And I still rely heavily on my faith. I think he'll bring me through with this too.

Interviewer: Okay. Okay. I'm a … I might come back … just … can you tell me how you view quality of life. What I mean quality of life … for some people, quality of life means being able to get up every day. And, and um, go to work every day, and um, um, got to work every day. And um, have good health or have good relationships with your families … good quality of life or a good relationship with God. Uh, not, not having getting up every day and not having to worry about certain things. Being able to pay your bills or whatever. There's a wide variety of ways you can um, describe quality of life. Okay? Can you tell me what quality of life means to you today.

1st Man: Well, um, it really means, uh, me being in good standing with my family. There ups and downs in my … and I think I love each of the sons and I thank God … and this helps … that helps … spiritually. Plus I love Him … Love Jesus … Jesus Christ. I love the combination of how it could be … I think.

Interviewer: When you say good standing with your family, what do you mean good standing?

1st Man: Um, really have sharing and caring … whenever ones in need. I can always depend upon them to come in to the rescue – come in to the rescue.

Interviewer: Um-hmm.

1st Man:	And that works … all of us have the same idea …
Interviewer:	Um-hmm.
1st Man:	… towards each other …
Interviewer:	Um-hmm.
1st Man:	… and that just about sums it up.

One-on-One Interview

Throughout my career, I have conducted interviews using focus group and one-on-one face-to-face formats. My preference is the one-on-one, face-to-face, semi-structured interview format. I have learned that during these types of interviews, I am able to engage with the participant and conduct a more in-depth exploration of the patient experience. I have found that participants are more open during one-on-one interviews than during focus group interviews. This preference for one-on-one interview formats is likely the result of my background and love of storytelling—the love to get the unexpected story. Even when I did conduct focus groups, I found myself conducting one-on-one follow-up interviews to get a story that was not possible in a group interview.

In the two examples below, I illustrate my experience with an information-rich interview and information-poor interview. In the first interview, in spite of my loaded interview questions, I was still able to get the story of how a cancer diagnosis affected the patient from the family members' perspective. This information-rich interview is likely the result of my telling the family member ahead of the interview what questions I planned to ask but also her motivation to be better able to support her family member through my research.

Notice the participant responses (cancer patient caregiver) in the information rich interview are not only lengthy following the interview question but focused on the topic with little to no probing. These information-rich responses could be attributed to the participant's desire to confide in an outsider about her caregiver experience but also to the unstructured approach I took to beginning the interview.

Example 5 Information Rich Interview

I: Interviewer
P: Participant
I: … same thing from you. If you could just start out talking to me about in your opinion how cancer has affected his life.
P: Ok.
I: Just whatever you want to tell me. Cause you know more about it.
P: Well um, we've been together probably about six months and um, when I first met [name], you know, he was um, he was on I guess a different medications that he's on, you know, it, it affects him. He's on this new medication now. When I first met him he wasn't on this medication where he, you know he gets, he can get real moody, ok. Now since he started taking the new medication now I forgot the name of it what he's taking, um, he's better, you know

he's um, when he takes it. A lot of times he gets mad at himself, you know he gets mad that he has to take the mediation every day and tells me and I try to make sure he took it. But he tells me you know I'm feeling fine, you know, I'm feeling fine and I don't need to take it, so a lot of times when he don't take it, you know, um, he's real moody. Like within the last six months um, we've separated four or five times you know, because of his attitude you know. It's a don't care attitude you know he'll say, you know, um, I'm dying anyway and you know stuff like that and um, or he'll say he don't want nobody to care about him. I guess he don't, he don't want nobody to worry about him. I don't know, but he, he a lot of times he tells me he don't want anyone to care about him and that was, from what I understood from him and his family, he's been through a lot, you know, with relationships, relationship problems um, where women used him or whatever. So at this point in his life it feels to me that he cant believe that there's someone that cares about him that, that would be there for him you know, no matter what, you know then he says um, he, he don't understand why he hadn't had that in his life, why it had to come now that he has the cancer, you know, that he doesn't he's going to be around for much longer you know, why at this point that, you know that somebody cares about him like that. And sometimes I don't believe, I love him with all my heart, you know and there's nothing that I wouldn't do for him and um, he would ask me why. You know he's always asking me why. You know he treats, sometimes he treats me like crap, you know, I leave and I come back and you know he doesn't understand why, I tell him I love you, I love you so much and I know he's a good person, you know he's a real good person. The cancer it, you know, it makes him, Edward is real moody with a lot of people. He doesn't, he doesn't have many friends at all and it's like he doesn't want to be bothered, you know. A lot of times, a lot of days when um, like when it's nice and stuff and I'll say, you know cause I don't work either, you know both of us are at home, um, most um, all day and I'll ask him, I'll say baby well lets get out and take a walk or something like that, you know, and you know he just likes to stay in bed a lot, you know at home and he's such a moody person, like if somebody went, if we go somewhere and somebody speak to him you know and he's like I don't want to speak to that person or, you know, he's just um, sometimes like the phone-the phone could ring and he gets mad because of the phone ringing, but yet he still want a phone, but he get mad because the phone rings. Somebody could knock at the door, you know and he's, he's just a moody person a lot of times, but um, when he takes his medication, um, that he's prescribed, the way that he's supposed to take it, you know this new medication that he's taking, when he takes that, that makes a big difference, that medication that he's taking.

I: Tell me about some of the things that he's, he's um, and I know some of this you already said, but tell me again about some of the things he's needed help with.

P: What do you mean?

I: What kinds of things he's needed help with, like taking him places he needs to go, maybe driving him or helping him get around.

P: Well yeah, well there's not a whole lot of places that he goes. You know, he comes down to his doctor's appointments and stuff and you know he um, um, you know we come down here on the bus or whatever, you know. His um, financial situation is stuck, you know he gets his social security check, his um check every month and stuff and um, I guess mainly the help is with like with the food, you know. Keeping food in the house from month to month you now because the bills aren't really that high, the rent is a fixed rent and stuff, our utilities are not really that high and stuff, you know. you know and then mainly, you know a lot of times, he'll be like you know he want to just get on the bus and ride and you know a lot of times he don't have bus money to do those things you know and he'll express to me about just doing things, just getting out sometimes you know and um, you know we just don't have the finances to do that, but.

I: What about um, in terms of getting information that you need about his cancer?

P: Oh we get, we get real good information especially down here, when we come down here, you know we get pamphlets and um, my son goes online and he's been online and he's gotten some information because um, first when [name] and I was together, we first started, when it started out and when he had these mood swings and stuff and you know I didn't know cause I've never been with um, somebody that has cancer or anything and you know it scared me that he was going to drop dead on me or whatever. It did until, you know because I didn't know. That's why I started coming down here with him to his appointments because when he- when we first got together and he'd come down here and I'd ask him you know well what did the doctor say and uh, he says I'm alright and you know now that's why I come so I can ask questions, ask the doctor questions because I don't know and I care about him and I need to know, you know, I want to know.

I: What about um, when he's worried about things, are there any things that you do to maybe distract him or keep him, his mind off of it?

P: When [name] is worried about something, I don't care what nobody says or whatever, if he's worried about something and a lot of times [name] don't share. He don't like to share his feelings or what he's worried about, you know, he'll say I'll work it out, I'll work it out and then he pushes me away, so he doesn't let me help him.

I: Is there anything that you do when he does that?

P: Well I used to get mad at him and um, just fuss at him, you know I just hound him about you know let me know, tell me what's going on, tell me what's going on, but um, I started just leaving him alone, I leave him alone, I found when I leave him alone he'll sit in one room; he likes to listen to music, you know, he's got a lot of music so um, he'll sit in there, he'll listen to his music and then I might sit in living room and watch tv or whatever until he comes around, so I found that's the most effective way because um, you know I keep hounding him and then – and sometimes he shares it with me you know, whatever is going on, sometimes he doesn't.

I: What about um, in terms of um, things that he's been responsible for like around the house or other things he might have been responsible for, even before he got diagnosed like um, like if there were chores around the house or stuff happening with his mother, or –

P: Well I don't know how he was, I don't know how he was before um, he got diagnosed, but um, now I mean he does most of the chores around the house. He does you know, now when like he gets mad at me or whatever, you know, that's when he really does chores. You know he's washing dishes, he do more around the house than I do, so you know he's really, really responsible around the house all the time.

I: Ok. Alright. Is there anything else that you can think of that I haven't thought to ask?

P: Um, I don't know if this is a um, anything about cancer patients, he uh, he's just overly clean or whatever, but have you ever heard of cancer patients liking to take baths all the time? Is that– I don't know, uh, I don't know if he thinks he's washing it away, I don't know, he takes, he takes a lot of baths.

I: Does he?

P: Yeah he takes about sometimes three, four into a bath, bubble bath, you know.

I: You know what, it may be calming. It calms him down maybe.

P: Yeah, that's probably is, you're probably right because sometimes when he's mad, you know I hear him in there running the water, yeah, yeah.

I: It must be something soothing about it.

P: Yeah, yeah, cause he, he in that tub all the time– a lot. Yeah I think you're right.

I: And I've heard that before.

P: Yeah he does, he's like three, four, sometimes five. He'll go in there –

I: Now you told me some, my next question is tell, just tell me you told me all the things he's needed help with, but which of those things do you think that you've been able to help more with and help less with and I can kind of hear, I hear what you're saying is those times when he kind of like goes off to his self when he gets like really moody or upset, that kind of thing, that's the times that you have the most problems trying to help him cause he's not –

P: Uh huh, yeah um. I can't, I don't know what to do to you know to calm him down with his, when he goes into his little moods except for, for leave him alone. A lot of times I don't want to you know, I want to be close to him and you know cause I want, like I said I care about him and I care about what's going on with him so um, you know I cant really do anything about that.

I: Does he, does he um, cause you're around him most, does he talk to anybody else about what he's going through?

P: No. No, nobody, no.

I: Ok. Sometimes um, sometimes people don't want to um, be a burden to the people that they love and care about the most.

P: Yeah.

I: Then they have stuff and they feel like if they talk to much it will cause that person to worry. What I call it is um, especially men, men – like men will protect their spouses, and you are like a spouse, but they will protect their spouses and their mothers and the way they do that is by not telling them, giving them a lot of information that will cause them to worry.

P: Yeah, well he always says, you know, he doesn't even tell– he'll talk to his dad on a daily basis and you know he really doesn't even let his dad know you know what's going on with him and stuff and you know he just tell me you know, he don't want anybody to worry about him, you know like um, sometimes and you know and like he might have um, pain from the scar, you know he had one of his kidneys removed and you know I don't hear him grunting or whatever, whatever, and I know he's in pain and you know I tell him, I say baby I say you know well why don't you take a pain pill, you know. Sometimes I can get him to take that pain pill and sometimes I can't you know, and so he will say don't worry about me, there's nothing wrong with me, I'm ok, I'm ok and I know he's not ok. But then sometimes I don't understand like [name] knows that he needs to take his medication on a daily basis. He knows that he's sick, he knows, you know he's got the cancer or whatever and he knows he needs to take it, but you know I don't understand why he wont just take it, you know, and he tells me I feel alright and sometimes I'll treat him like a baby, you know. I get up and I you know put coffee on and I make sure to give him his pills you know, becuase sometimes if I don't do it he wont take it. If he's feeling alright he wont take it you know, and that I don't understand. I just, and he knows his blood pressure is up and you know he has, he starts having headaches and I told him, I say baby have you taken your medication? Oh no I feel alright. You know, I – he's thick headed, I don't understand it.

I: My last question is – you know what I want to ask you to because last time he talks a lot about God brought him through, God, and I hear that everytime he has hard times.

P: Yeah he knows, [name] um, he spent a lot of time, um a couple years homeless right before he got um, sick. And um, from what I understand, I think it was two years, well first of all he went through a bad marriage and you know it was um, like I said it was kind of a he said she abused him or whatever, but it was a real bad marriage where it was a one sided love and you know, he was just staying and staying and staying, and then he became homeless for a couple of years and um, when he got– actually when he got sick, he was homeless. He passed out on the sidewalk. He said he was doing some kind of um, getting ready to go to a labor pool or whatever and um, and right now he's um, he's in – we're in a comfortable apartment and everything and you know he's always saying you know God, God brought me a long way. I got a roof over my head, you know and I might not have what I want to eat, but you know I got food and you know I'm not out there, every time when we see a homeless person, you know, he says I'm not out there in the streets or anything like that and then he says God brought you to me, you know and so he's, he's just – he ain't told me that one in a long time though (giggles).

I: Um, I'm, in my next study, cause you were in the one I'm in now, that I'm doing now, but my next study I want to do something to help like especially with the part about um, them not wanting to talk about what they're going through and not wanting to share, um, a lot of times even with, I mean he's not that, that old, but even you know with older, older than him, they have things that they need help with or they're having problems you know or whatever and they don't want to share it, but they might share it with a healthcare professional or somebody like me. And so I want to design a study, this is what I'm thinking, that I would design a study and that I could talk to maybe Edward and maybe he might share some things with me. Then I could help family members or whoever they're close to, to better support them because then I'm kind of relieving that –

P: Yeah that would be great, you know because sometimes I, you know I get frustrated you know cause I get mad with him because he wont let me know, you know, what's going on and I – sometimes I feel useless, you know sometimes and he don't want to share and you know like I said I care about him and I care about what's bothering him and you know he's – I'll take care of it, you don't need to worry about it. Yes I do need to worry about it, you know, but he can't seem to see that. But yeah that would be a splendid idea, yes.

I: Anything else that you could tell me that would help me?

P: Uh, I think we about covered it.

I: Ok, now if you think of anything, you know like anything after this is over even down the road or whatever, you know how to find me.

P: Yeah I sure do. I have your card.

I: You can call me. This has been very helpful to me, very helpful.

P: Ok.

In the example below [referred to as Information Poor], I was not able to get this participant to share details of his illness experience or his experience with bereavement. There could have been several reasons for this: My lack of skill with probing, my discomfort with silence [I did not give him time to process the question], he really did not want to do the interview but did not want to say no, or maybe his experience with the deaths of his wife and grandson did not affect him emotionally as I expected.

For this information-poor interview, I could have tried a second interview at a different time of day, with an interviewer of the same gender, or in the presence of a family member that might have encouraged him to tell his story. Unfortunately, for this project, I didn't have the resources for a second interview.

Example 6 Information Poor Interview

Transcript for Subject 52 Interview

Ten Minutes, Forty Seconds

Dr. Hamilton: "Okay. What's your age?"

S52: "Uh, seventy-eight."

Dr. Hamilton: "Okay. And years in school?"

S52: "I went to the ninth grade."

Dr. Hamilton: "Okay. And have you always been Baptist?"

S52: "Yeah, mhmm."

Dr. Hamilton: "Okay. You grew up here in Black Mountain?"

S52: "Yeah."

Dr. Hamilton: "Okay. And what's been the most stressful thing for you; you lost your wife—what year was that?"

S52:	"1959, on March the 18th when she died."
Dr. Hamilton:	"Now it wasn't 1959 … 1999?"
S52:	"No, 1959. Oh, when she died?"
Dr. Hamilton:	"When she died."
S52:	"1999."
Dr. Hamilton:	"1999."
S52:	"Around the time that I got married."
Dr. Hamilton:	"Okay, and then your grandson.
S52:	"Yeah, that was—"
Dr. Hamilton:	"I was following that in the paper."
S52:	"The 28th of May."
Dr. Hamilton:	"That was this year. Now what kinds of things do you see the doctor for?"
S52:	"Well, uh—I've got a … and high blood. I guess that's it."
Dr. Hamilton:	"And how long has it been since you lost your—is your sight completely gone?"
S52:	"Yeah. 1974."
Dr. Hamilton:	"You wanna just go on ahead and talk your favorite songs, and scriptures that helped you get through, uh, when you lost your wife and with your grandson? You have any favorite scriptures?"
S52:	"Well, one … I'll say Job was favorite scripture."
Dr. Hamilton:	"Okay."
S52:	"I can't have … too much reading."
Dr. Hamilton:	"Okay. But you remember the book of Job when you were younger or you like to hear people when they talk about it?"
S52:	" … I'll tell you when I started in 1985."
Dr. Hamilton:	"Uh huh."
S52:	"I had a lady—there's a lady and, uh—where we worked at … she was reading the Bible … and she started discussing the Bible with me then."
Dr. Hamilton:	"Oh, okay—on the job? Where was this?"
S52:	"On the … in Nashville."
Dr. Hamilton:	"Ohhhh! Okay. Alright, and so your favorite one was Job. Do you remember kind of which—what part of Job that you really liked?"
S52:	"It started all the way from the front. We didn't get to finish it because she got married and left before we finished."
Dr. Hamilton:	"Okay. But at church—do you ever go to bible study?"
S52:	"Every Wednesday."
Dr. Hamilton:	"That's what I thought. So what's your favorite scriptures from bible study that's helped you get through?"
S52:	"Well I think it was many of them but I can't—"
Dr. Hamilton:	"—But you know you like Job."
S52:	"Yeah, mhmm."
Dr. Hamilton:	"What is it you like about the story of Job?"
S52:	"Well, uh—well, he lost everything."
Dr. Hamilton:	"Okay … do you think about your life in relation to Job?"

S52: "Well, some ways I do."
Dr. Hamilton: "How is that?"
S52: "Well, I felt like when I lost my wife … then, uh, I lost my grandson … "
Dr. Hamilton: " … And what about, uh … when you think about Job and what he went through and what you've had to go through, um—how do you feel inside when you think about that?"
S52: "Well, that's a hard thing to say."
Dr. Hamilton: "Uh huh."
S52: "Most likely you feel like you're all alone, you know."
Dr. Hamilton: "Uh huh."
S52: " … but, uh, you think back—you ain't alone, you're just—that this is running through your mind … "
Dr. Hamilton: "Uh huh. Well, what helps you when you start feeling like you're all alone?"
S52: "Just say a prayer and that's it."
Dr. Hamilton: "So what do you ask God to do for you when you–?"
S52: "Just to help me get through it."
Dr. Hamilton: "And does that seem to help?"
S52: "Yeah."
Dr. Hamilton: "How often do you find yourself feeling like you're all alone?"
S52: "Well, uh—it's—it varies."
Dr. Hamilton: "Yeah."
S52: "I'd say it varies … "
Dr. Hamilton: "Okay, alright. Do you have any, like, favorite songs that helps you get through?"
S52: "Yes."
Dr. Hamilton: "What's some of your favorite."
S52: " … singing one last night, uh … 'Tell the Angels I'm Coming'—"
Dr. Hamilton: "Ohhhh! I don't know that one. How does that one go? I don't know that one … "
S52: (**Lyrics**)
Dr. Hamilton: "Ohhh! How does it go …? You know the tune to it?"
S52: "I don't know the tune to it. All I know is the song."
Dr. Hamilton: "But you sing it in choir … Is there another favorite one you like?"
S52: "I like one my uncle used to sing a long time ago: 'Will the Circle Be Unbroken.'
Dr. Hamilton: "Your uncle over here? Uncle (name omit)?"
S52: "No … "
Dr. Hamilton: "—'Will the Circle Be Unbroken'—I know that song. And you used to hear him sing it?"
S52: "Yeah, I used to hear him sing it all the time."
Dr. Hamilton: "And why do you—do you know why you like that one?"
S52: "No, I just like this that's all."
Dr. Hamilton: "—Just that—does it remind you of him?"
S52: "Yeah."

Dr. Hamilton:	"Okay … any more songs you can think of that you really like that you can remember from a long time ago? When you're singing in the choir do y'all still, like—you still like to sing those old songs?"
S52:	"Yes, but now they don't sing those old songs like that."
Dr. Hamilton:	"What do you think about that?"
S52:	"What?"
Dr. Hamilton:	"Them not singing them old songs?"
S52:	" … I like the old ones; you get more feeling than the old ones than you do these new ones."
Dr. Hamilton:	"Do you understand? Some people sat they don't—"
S52:	"Well, you don't understand all these new ones … "
Dr. Hamilton:	"The words? Yeah, that's what I heard people say. But y'all still sing the old ones don't you?"
S52:	"Oh yeah.
Dr. Hamilton:	"In the choir—the old ones that we grew up knowing."
S52:	"Yeah, mhmm."
Dr. Hamilton:	"Are they hymns?—or some of them are hymns, some of them are—"
S52:	"Some of them are hymns, some of them are something else."
Dr. Hamilton:	"Uh huh. Mhmm. Okay, that's all I have."
S52:	"Yeah."
Dr. Hamilton:	"That wasn't so bad, was it?"
S52:	"That wasn't bad; I thought that was gonna be bad."
Dr. Hamilton:	"You thought it was gonna be bad? Naww."

Structure of Interview Questions (Structured, Unstructured, Semi-Structured)

The structured interview questions. During data collection, I generally start with structured questions such as demographics or closed-ended, fixed response questions, I then move to structured or semi-structured, then open-ended interview questions. I start with structured questions for a couple reasons. Structured questions help to break the ice, establish rapport, and help me to get a feel for the way the participant uses language to express themselves (Merriam & Tisdel, 2016). Getting a feel for language used during the structured interview gives me insight into words or phrases I need to use when I am asking semi-structured interview questions. A final reason to start with the structured questions is that if for some reason, I am not able to complete the interview, I will have the demographics and can use whatever data I was able to collect.

A suggestion about the structured interview and demographics: I collect as much data as I possible to describe the participant and possibly any factors that could influence responses to interview questions. During explorations about social support, I collect the usual age, gender, education, employment, marital status, and income but also information about religious affiliation, geographical location, state grew up in, and how long they have lived in current community, city, and state. I always ask for participants to self-identify their racial/ethnic group as I never assume this information based on physical characteristics.

Below is an example of a structured questionnaire that I have used to capture the demographics of older African American cancer survivors. The structured questions are detailed but provide a broader description of the factors likely to shape the social support experiences of the interviewee.

Example 7 Structured Interview Questions

TELL US ABOUT YOU

1. How old are you? age
   Age: ☐☐ years

   Date of birth ☐☐/☐☐/19☐☐
   mm dd yy

2. Are you female or male? gender
   Female.................... 1 ☐
   Male.......................2 ☐

3. What is your race? race
   (CHECK all that apply)
   African American, Black, or Negro...1 ☐
   American Indian/ Alaska Native.........2 ☐
   Asian/Pacific Islander........................ 3 ☐
   White ....4 ☐
   Other..5 ☐
   If other, write in________________

4. What do you consider your racial, ethnic or cultural background or heritage? This may be the countries or regions your ancestors were from. ethnicit

   ____

   ____

5. How much does this background affect your everyday life? backgrd
   Not at all..................................0 ☐
   A little ....1 ☐
   Some ....2 ☐
   Quite a bit..................................3 ☐
   A great deal ....4 ☐

6. What is the highest grade in school that you completed? educatio
   Completed 6th grade or less......................1 ☐
   Junior high school (7th - 9th grade).....2 ☐
   Partial high school (10th - 11th grade)..3 ☐
   High school graduate or GED....................4 ☐
   Partial college training ....5 ☐
   Completed college.......................................6 ☐
   Graduate professional training................7 ☐
   Other________________________............8 ☐

7. What kind of work have you done most of your working life? typejob

   ____

   ____

8. What is your current marital status? marstat
   Married.........................1 ☐
   Widowed.......................2 ☐
   Divorced ....3 ☐
   Separated ....4 ☐
   Never married..............5 ☐
   Partnered ....6 ☐

9. Counting yourself, how many people live in your household? livehous
   ____☐☐____people

10. Do you have children under age 18 living in your household or for whom you have responsibilities? age18
    No..................0
    Yes 1

    If YES, numage18
    10a. How many? __________
    10b. About how many hours per week do you spend in caring for or supervising these children? _____ hrs/wk? Hrswkage18

TELL US ABOUT YOU

11. What state/country were you born in? born
____

12. How many years have you lived in the city or town where you currently reside? ☐☐ yearscty

13. What is your religious affiliation? affiliat

Baptist....................................1 ☐
Buddhist...................................2 ☐
Catholic....................................3 ☐

Episcopal..................................4 ☐
Holiness...................................5 ☐
Jewish......................................6 ☐

Lutheran...................................7 ☐
Methodist..................................8 ☐
Mormon (LDL).............................9 ☐

Muslim......................................10 ☐
Non-Denominational ....11 ☐
Pentecostal..............................12 ☐

Presbyterian.............................13 ☐
Protestant.................................14 ☐
Unitarian Universalist..............15 ☐

Do not have any affiliation....16 ☐
Other...17 ☐
If other, write in______________

14. What is the total amount of your yearly household income before taxes? Please include money from jobs, net income from a business or farm, dividends, interest, net income from rent, social security, gifts, and any other money income. yrincome

Yearly Household Income

$1- $2,499..................................1 ☐

$ 2 ,500- $4,999.........................2 ☐

$5,000-$9,999 ....3 ☐

$10,000-$14,999.........................4 ☐

$15,000-$19,999.........................5 ☐

$20,000-$24,999.........................6 ☐

$25,000-$29,999.........................7 ☐

$30,000-$34,999.........................8 ☐

$35,000-$39,999.........................9 ☐

$40,000-$44,999.........................10 ☐

$45,000-$49,999.........................11 ☐

$50 ,000-$74,999 ....12 ☐

$75,000-$99,999.........................13 ☐

$100,000 and more ....14 ☐

The unstructured interview question. I have used the unstructured interview question when I was wanting to learn about a patient experience with no knowledge of how to proceed (Maxwell, 2013; Merriam & Tisdel, 2016). The unstructured interview question is used to initiate the interview. After introductions and explaining the purpose of the study, I start by explaining in a language understood by the interviewee how I would like to begin. For example, "Let's start with when you were diagnosed with cancer, tell me how you felt." This unstructured question is helpful for several reasons.

The time when they were diagnosed and feeling associated with that time is likely information they are able to recall. The feelings experienced at the time of a cancer diagnosis are ones not likely shared with others, and the interview is the opportunity to express those feelings. See below for an example of ways in which I have used the unstructured interview question.

The semi-structured interview question. The interview question that is somewhat structured, while permitting flexibility to capture emerging themes with input from the interviewee is the most frequently used in my qualitative research projects. The semi-structured interview question starts with an interview guide with open-ended questions that can be added, deleted, or tweaked based on the flow of the conversation and need to follow unanticipated lines of inquiry. Although there is no specific number of questions required for the interview guide for semi-structured interview questions, I always recommend a small number. This small number of questions

Example 8 Unstructured Interview Questions

First Example Question: Can you talk some about, how, you changed the way you saw yourself from, before the cancer diagnosis?

Second Example Question: Could you talk about how, what was the image you had of yourself when you were told that you had a cancer diagnosis?

Participant: Um, I think at first, I was, like, feeling guilty. Um, I was thinking … Like, I think at a point in time, in the beginning, I was feeling as if, like, "Is this punishment for something that I've done?" Um, like, karma or something like that. And then, like, also, um, my mom, um, as you know, was diagnosed, like, maybe a year or so prior to my diagnosis. And, like, I felt like I wasn't as supportive as I should be because it was very emotional for me, like, while she was going through her situation. So, it was like … It was just hard for me to, like, be around 'cause I just would always just break down crying. So, I didn't– I don't feel like I did what I should've done as far as being supportive in that role. Um, and so, I– I had a lot of guilt when I was diagnosed, like, "You should've stepped up more for your mom. You should've done this. You should've done that," especially, like, when I went through it and all of the, like, struggles and stuff that I had in that moment. Um, so yeah, that was like the image that I would say, like, feeling a sense of … Like questioning, like, "Why?" Like, "Why me? What did I do to deserve this?"

prevents the interviewer from overpowering the interviewee with a set of predetermined questions that silences the voice of the participant. Generally, the research questions guiding my qualitative projects are mostly exploratory in nature with very little evidence on the topic. For these topics, I sometimes start with an unstructured question and structure them as the interview progresses and as I learn more about the topic from the participant.

See below for an example of ways in which I have used the semi-structured interview question.

Example 9 Semi-Structured Interview Questions

I: What about um, when he's worried about things, are there any things that you do to maybe distract him or keep him, his mind off of it?

P: When [name] is worried about something, I don't care what nobody says or whatever, if he's worried about something and a lot of times [name] don't share. He don't like to share his feelings or what he's worried about, you know, he'll say I'll work it out, I'll work it out and then he pushes me away, so he doesn't let me help him.

I: Is there anything that you do when he does that?

P: Well I used to get mad at him and um, just fuss at him, you know I just hound him about you know let me know, tell me what's going on, tell me what's going on, but um, I started just leaving him alone, I leave him alone, I found when I leave him alone he'll sit in one room; he likes to listen to music, you know, he's got a lot of music so um, he'll sit in there, he'll listen to his music and then I might sit in living room and watch tv or whatever until he comes around, so I found that's the most effective way because um, you know I keep hounding him and then – and sometimes he shares it with me you know, whatever is going on, sometimes he doesn't.

I: What about um, in terms of um, things that he's been responsible for like around the house or other things he might have been responsible for, even before he got diagnosed like um, like if there were chores around the house or stuff happening with his mother, or –

P: Well I don't know how he was, I don't know how he was before um, he got diagnosed, but um, now I mean he does most of the chores around the house. He does you know, now when like he gets mad at me or whatever, you know, that's when he really does chores. You know he's washing dishes, he do more around the house than I do, so you know he's really, really responsible around the house all the time.

I: Ok. Alright. Is there anything else that you can think of that I haven't thought to ask?

P: Um, I don't know if this is a um, anything about cancer patients, he uh, he's just overly clean or whatever, but have you ever heard of cancer patients liking to take baths all the time? Is that– I don't know, uh, I don't know if he thinks he's washing it away, I don't know, he takes, he takes a lot of baths.

Conducting Follow-Up Interviews

I request follow-up interviews for several reasons. First the interview is taking longer than the agreed upon time. During the interview, I closely monitor the time and once I determine that more than 45 minutes will be needed to obtain responses to the questions, I will request a second, follow-up interview. The second interview for this first reason allows me to complete the interview in a deliberate and calm, not rushed pace.

The second reason for a follow-up interview is to permit me additional time to explore areas or topics that I failed to pursue during the interview. Earlier in my research career, there were times that I was so focused on the next question or taking notes that I failed to hear and subsequently follow up on a critical thought expressed by the participants. I generally recognize this omission after the interview and when I am reviewing the typed transcript. Having the participants' permission to recontact for a second, follow-up interview permits a follow-up of these topics.

The third reason to request a follow-up interview is when topics emerge in subsequent interviews that I would like to explore their relevance among participants in earlier interviews. In one case, the third and fourth participant described God as a source of social support which had not emerged in earlier interviews. Again, when I have permission from the IRB and the participant for a second, follow-up interview, I am able to explore the emerging topics with earlier participants.

I always include in the IRB application whether I might return to participants for follow-up interviews, and a statement for this request is included in the consent form. I also request follow-up interviews from participants during the first interview. I tell them the reason for the second, follow-up interview and whether it can be in person or over the telephone. See below for a section of a transcript where I am explaining the purpose of this second, follow-up interview with a participant.

Example 10 Follow-Up Interview Request

PI: So basically, I'm doing this extra interview 'cause I want to learn more about those things that are bothersome or stressful for African American cancer patients. Okay?

PI: … and like I said, when we get closer to like, maybe like 10:40 or something like that. If I look like we got a-, a ways to go, I'm gonna stop it and then we will schedule another time to finish up 'cause I'd rather for you to be able to take your time and talk …

GC: Mm, okay.

PI: … um, even if we have to do it over two times. Okay?

GC: Okay.

Closing the Interview

When closing the interview, remember to never turn off the recording device until you are completely out of the door. I cannot tell you how frequently I have turned off the recorder only to have the participant give me additional information that I wish I would have had recorded.

Example 11 Closing the Interview

Thank you very much for sharing your experience and opinions with us. Your responses will be very helpful to us in getting a good idea of what types of help or support are of benefit to others with cancer.

If you would like us to send you a summary of the study findings, please call Dr. Hamilton at 404 xxx-xxxx.

Thank you again for your participation!

At closing, I thank the participant for their time, remind them of the importance of their story, make sure they have their incentive (given prior to the interview), and remind the participant of the possibility for an additional second follow-up interview. I also make sure they have my contact information in case they have additional information for their interview or just want to follow up with an outcome of the study. I always leave my cell phone and email, and let them know they are welcome to reach out directly to me at any time. The next example illustrates a written closing statement that might be included on some document that stays with the participant after the interview.

A Note on Taking Notes

Qualitative methods scholars frequently recommend taking notes (field notes) during the interview and even after the interview. I have used field notes to document any observations that may supplement any descriptions of the participants either individually or as a sample. I may take notes on when and how a participant was recruited, when and where they were interviewed, the length of the interview, whether any family members were present during the interview, and any closing thoughts I may have about the participant and any interesting comments made during the interview. Immediately after the interview or focus group, I will spend some time to record any field notes in a notebook I keep with my recording devices. I may also actually record my field notes for transcription for electronic storage with the typed interview.

Conclusion

In this chapter, I discussed topics to aid with the actual interview. I have discussed my experiences with the focus group vs the one-on-one in-person interview and included a discussion on the pros and cons of each type of interview with exemplars of information-rich vs information-poor interviews. In the second section of this chapter, I discuss the structured, unstructured, and semi-structured interview questions with examples of each. The remaining sections are discussions focused on when to conduct follow-up interviews, how to close the interview, and the usefulness of recording notes on the interview. In the next chapter, I discuss strategies to maintain rigor during the interview with examples from my SDOH research conducted among an underserved population.

References

Maxwell, J. A. (2013). *Qualitative Research Design: An Interactive Approach*. Thousand Oaks, CA, Sage Publications, Inc.
Merriam, S. B. and E. J. Tisdel. (2016). *Qualitative Research: A Guide to Design and Implementation*. San Francisco, CA, Jossey-Bass.
Morgan, D. L. (2019). *Basic and Advanced Focus Groups*. Thousand Oaks, CA, Sage Publishing.

8 Rigor in Qualitative Research

In this chapter, I discuss the usefulness or appropriateness of strategies to achieve rigor when using qualitative methods in SDOH research. These strategies include prolonged engagement and thick, rich description; negative case analysis; peer review or briefing; clarifying researcher bias; member checking; investigator triangulation and inter-coder reliability and the uses of these strategies among underrepresented populations. I omitted the discussion of audit trail in the previous publication on rigor but include it in this chapter.

Qualitative methods are frequently used to explore issues of relevance to underrepresented populations. Among community-dwelling populations, qualitative methods have been used to garner input to develop or tailor interventions that are culturally relevant (Garner & Faucher, 2014; Holliday et al., 2018) to improve participation rates in intervention studies (Bowers et al., 2017; Buseh et al., 2017) to better understand influences on outcomes of faith-based health programs (Stewart, 2015), and to develop and adapt instruments that are appropriate (Lee et al., 2015). Included in research reports using qualitative methods are discussions of strategies that are widely used and accepted as necessary to achieve rigor with qualitative methods. The list of strategies frequently includes prolonged engagement, audit trail, member checking, peer debriefing, triangulation, and inter-coder reliability (Maxwell, 2013). Strategies to achieve rigor may be inappropriately applied in qualitative research and treated similar to a checklist or a standard for quality regardless of the intent of the research (Morse, 2018).

In this chapter, I reflect on and critique the usefulness and appropriateness of strategies to achieve rigor in qualitative research that I have conducted among underrepresented minority and rural populations. The philosophical positioning of my program of research with African Americans is grounded in the social constructionism paradigm (Guba & Lincoln, 1994; Schwandt, 2000). Social constructivism aims to discover the experiences of individuals as lived, taking into consideration the cultural and historical norms of a population (Guba & Lincoln, 1994). Guided by this philosophical stance, the overall goal of my research with this population is to give voice to the social support experiences among older African Americans with life-threatening illness, to capture the strengths of this population, and to conduct research using a process that is trustworthy and authentic. However, I realize that I have been blindly using a prescribed list of strategies to enhance rigor was blindly used without thought to their relevance or appropriateness. Therefore, in this critique, I reflect on and evaluate the strategies used to enhance the trustworthiness of the qualitative studies that I have conducted.

Prolonged engagement, persistent observation, and thick, rich description. In combination, these strategies are generally used to ensure that the findings of a qualitative study

DOI: 10.4324/9781003598916-8

are "data rich," trustworthy (Morse, 2015), and transferable (Creswell, 1994). The attainment of thick, rich data include a consideration for quality time spent with participants, developing trusting relationships between interviewer/interviewee, research burden, and recruitment of a sample that is adequate and appropriate for the purpose of the study (Morse, 2015). These strategies are discussed in the following sections.

Quality time spent and interviewer/interviewee trusting relationships. In the conduct of research with African Americans, time to generate data that is information-rich largely depended on quality time and the development of trusting relationships between interviewer/interviewee. Scholars have characterized African American populations as distrustful of healthcare systems and research (Corbie-Smith et al., 2012; Haynes-Maslow et al., 2014). This mistrust has been attributed to the abuses from the U.S. Public Health Service Untreated Syphilis Study at Tuskegee or Henrietta Lacks studies where the human rights of African Americans were violated (Haynes-Maslow et al., 2014). The Tuskegee Syphilis Study was a project conducted and funded by the U.S. government funded that violated the human rights of African American men (Ponterotto, 2010; White, 2003). The purpose of the Tuskegee study was to study the natural history of syphilis; however, men in this study were never informed that they had syphilis and they were also denied treatment long after a cure became available. Henrietta Lacks' human rights were violated when U.S. scientists used her cancer cells in research without consent (Gamble, 2014). However, these characterizations of African Americans as fatalistic and distrustful based on these racial injustices are likely to reflect stereotypes rather than reality (Easterling, 2014).

Scholars have reported that underrepresented populations are not necessarily fatalistic or even aware of these high-profile racial injustices (Easterling, 2014). Rather, the illness experience and access to health care for African Americans is likely influenced by a history of reliance on home remedies that stem from low wages, lack of insurance, and the limited access to healthcare practitioners and facilities in their towns (Behringer & Krishnan, 2011; Coyne et al., 2006). The expressed distrust among African Americans can be attributed to personal experiences with racial discrimination through the receipt of poor health care (Behringer & Krishnan, 2011).

Quality time and trusting relationships needed for thick, rich data among underrepresented minority populations consist of a variety of strategies. In addition to ensuring that participants are informed of study procedures, a significant amount of time should be spent interacting with participants to develop a trusting interviewer/interviewee relationship. Quality time can be enhanced through listening to participants' stories in an unhurried and relaxed manner. Also important to quality time are efforts to convey to the participants that what they have to say is important and understood. I have been fortunate to have interviewed older African Americans in the 80- to 90-year-old range. During these interviews, I was extremely grateful to have spent my formative years in a small rural town which provided me the skill set to understand the vernacular used among this population. Follow-up or probing questions used during interviews were "Tell me more about that" to encourage participants to continue a storyline important to them and to provide assurance that their stories were valued.

Trust in interviewer-interviewee relationships can never be assumed. Although I grew up in one of the rural towns from which I was attempting to access and had visited church congregations in neighboring towns, I had not maintained ties with these individuals. I could not assume that being African American or a former member of the community would make the conduct of research among this racially and ethnically similar population easier (Fryer et al., 2016). I had moved away from this geographical region years ago to attend college, and since that time, I have only occasionally returned for short visits. The development of a trusting relationship was critical to open dialogue during interviews and to elicit quality data (Dale et al., 2017).

A primary strategy that I have used to enhance a trusting interviewer/interviewee relationship includes those that connected me to the population through kinship (close and extended family) ties (Presley, 2013). For example, when recruiting participants, I frequently reveal to participants my affiliations with family members in the area which I am recruiting. I am cautious with sharing my religious affiliation since this information could inhibit open conversation related to expected social behaviors related to religious doctrine. I share with participants my academic qualifications to conduct the research; affiliations with educational institutions; publications and church newsletters showcasing my research; and assure participants of my commitment to improving health outcomes among the population. As a show of respect for the cultural traditions and religious holidays of the population, recruitment and data collection is never scheduled to occur during the Sabbath and any other religious or major holiday associated with family gatherings. Especially important to a trusting interviewer/interviewee relationship is a show of respect for their values and personal space by wearing appropriate attire and salutations of the interviewees. Also, important is addressing participants as Mr. or Mrs. last name, casual business dress, and punctuality in appointments. Finally, conveying a sincere interest in the issues or stories of the population is critical. I frequently listened to stories that veered away from the intended focus of the research. The participant has benefited from the ability to express themselves and I as a scientist have benefited from learning about unanticipated topics or issues.

In addition to a consideration for developing trusting interviewer/interviewee relationships, quality of time spent during interviewers must consider the quality of time spent and the burden of the research on participants. Strategies to enhance rigor should include considerations for low reading levels or when participants are experiencing illness symptoms such as pain or fatigue. Thus, generating quality data may require interview times that are brief, focused, and when participants are well rested. Rather than conduct one long interview, I incorporate into the study design the collection of data over one or more interviews of shorter durations. A follow-up interview is sometimes needed to add information participants had forgotten to mention during the first interview or topics that I failed to address. The strategy of short and more frequent interviews minimizes the burden of the interview on the participant. It also permits the interviewee more time to respond to thought-provoking questions, and allowing the interviewer to follow up or probe on topics possibly missed during the initial interview. Understandably, this strategy is not feasible or even necessary for all studies but it would likely enhance rigor in studies that require the sampling of seriously ill participants.

A final strategy for building trusting relationships with interviewees is to permit them to have input into how their stories will or will not be used. In the consent forms or fact sheets, I inform participants that I may use their stories in future intervention studies or to educate students, I also elicit participant feedback. Participants have reported their opposition to having their stories appear on social media but instead provided input into specific ways they would like their stories used to benefit the community.

Sampling adequacy and appropriateness. In qualitative reports, adequacy of sample size is generally determined by whether the data were saturated rather than some a priori number based on statistical power analysis (Morse, 2015). Data saturation implies that during the process of sampling and analysis, no new information appears, and theoretical concepts are well-developed (Morse, 2015). Although generalizability is not the focus of qualitative inquiry, another consideration for sampling adequacy is whether the participants enrolled in the study are representative of a larger population or at a minimum capture the range of variables known to influence a particular experience (Merriam & Tisdel, 2016).

African Americans in any geographical region are not homogeneous. Therefore, sampling strategies should include a consideration for a range of demographic characteristics and variables that possibly influence participant experiences and therefore sampling adequacy (Carminati, 2018). For example, when the focus of my research was to understand the social support experiences not emphasized in existing research, sampling strategies included a consideration for demographic and theoretical variations analytically important to coping and social support experiences (Hamilton & Sandelowski, 2004; Lazarus & Folkman, 1984). During the conduct of research with African Americans, I purposefully recruited participants who varied on demographic variables (person factors) i.e. gender, income, education, and marital status (Hamilton et al., 2013a, 2013b, 2016, 2017). In addition to demographic variations, I also purposefully recruited participants based on theoretical (situational) variations. For purposes of this social support research, situational variations were conceptualized as clinical variables (i.e., type and stage of cancer). These variables served as markers for illness severity that could possibly influence one's appraisal of their illness as threatening or not and subsequently their social support experience (Hamilton & Sandelowski, 2004).

Variations in demographics and clinical variables promote expanded understandings of the patterns of supportive exchanges among network members as well as the types of social support involved in those exchanges (Hamilton & Sandelowski, 2004). As interviews progressed, demographic variations were expanded to include type of stressful life event, proximity to family (whether individuals lived alone or not), and geographic location (rural vs. urban geographic locations) (Hamilton et al., 2013a, 2013b, 2016, 2017). Finally, during data analysis, those additional variations that became apparent were prominent cultural influences that included racism, religion, and spirituality. These cultural variations were important considerations in illuminating the influences on trusting relationships and supportive experiences among participants in previous research, but also the future direction of subsequent qualitative studies that I have conducted. Important considerations when conducting research among African Americans and any minority population, therefore, is to recognize the diversity with respect to demographic, situational, and cultural influences on a particular experience. This diversity is essential to accurately portray the voice of this population.

Sampling appropriateness is not always immediately obvious when the focus of the research question is relatively unknown. Initial segue into communities that are rural or isolated or even unknown to the researcher may appear highly unorganized. Recruitment in these communities may begin with a combination of convenient volunteers known to the researcher and snowballing. Once recruitment is underway, it will become clearer who has the desired experience to answer interview questions, and as patterns emerge from the findings, sampling strategies may be refined. Revisions are frequently necessary to capture the desired experiences that generate information-rich data focused on the topic.

Negative case analysis. In qualitative inquiry, the tendency is to focus on identifying and understanding those cases with quotes that can be readily identified as connected to the topic and frequently occurring and to discard negative cases with quotes that appear infrequently or are inconsistent with the overall study purpose (Morse, 2015). However, these negative cases might be critical to understanding subpopulation differences and the "whole" of the experience being studied (Morse, 2015). In an earlier study that focused on the social support experiences of older African American cancer patients, one negative or outlying case was of a survivor who described bargaining with God for survival (Hamilton & Sandelowski, 2004). Although it would have been optimal to fully explore whether bargaining with God had been an experience with other participants during data collection, the reality was that this exemplar quote was not apparent until I was in the process of coding the data for a manuscript. During recruitment, I had only requested a one-time interview, so there was no opportunity to return for an additional interview. Rather than discard the quote as not relevant, I included this quote in the reported findings and explored whether this was an experience of participants in subsequent research. Interestingly, the experience of bargaining with God emerged more frequently during interviews among younger African Americans (Hamilton et al., 2018). In subsequent projects, I learned that it was not uncommon for younger African Americans to bargain with God or to even express anger with God. However, I would not have learned this had I not pursued this outlying theme in future research.

Peer debriefing and researcher bias. Peer review and debriefing are strategies that, when used, might assist the researcher in managing interviewer bias or bringing clarity to the conceptualization of the experience and related themes. I have over 25 years of research expertise with explorations of social and cultural factors influencing health outcomes among rural and community-dwelling African Americans using qualitative methods, yet I use peer debriefing to manage interviewer bias and to assist with conceptual clarity during data analysis and manuscript writing. For peer debriefing, I have collaborated with African American cancer survivors and caregivers, racially diverse healthcare providers (oncologists, nurses, social workers), and theologians with expertise in religion and culture. I selected these individuals for their clinical expertise with the population, expertise on the topic of race and religion, and their ability to provide an additional lens to the findings, conclusions, and/or implications. More importantly, it is the representation of the target population as key collaborators. These individuals participate in the research from the point of study design, giving input into interview questions, interpretation, and dissemination of findings.

Another benefit of peer debriefing is to manage the tendency for bias created from overlooking the obvious or lacking a neutral stance on findings that emerged during interviews similar to that reported in ethnographic research (LeCompte & Schensul, 1999). For example, since I had grown up attending a Southern Baptist Church where singing and testimonies were common, it was difficult for me initially to see the uniqueness of this practice or relevance to health outcomes outside of that environment. However, peer debriefing with racially diverse collaborators helped to clarify my thinking of the novelty of this spiritual practice as a type of complementary and alternative therapy in patient care. A second bias originated from my tendency to primarily focus on the positives of spirituality on health outcomes. Although the overwhelming majority of participants in these completed studies recalled positive experiences in the use of spiritual practices as mental health-promoting strategies; there were interviews with participants during which the recall of a religious song evoked sad memories of the death of a loved one. And, as mentioned previously, it was not uncommon for younger adults to express their anger at God for allowing their suffering. Peer debriefing with a diverse team of collaborators encourages an awareness of bias and the need to be open to positive and negative aspects of spiritual practices.

Finally, peer review is used to manage interviewer bias inherent in the selection of interview questions. Interview questions generally originate from investigators who are sensitized by their own experiences or through literature which results in a tendency to overlook issues of importance to the population (LeCompte & Schensul, 1999). Years ago, research focused on African American cancer survivors was extremely limited and conceptualizations of social support had not incorporated diverse perspectives of the Divine and God as a source of support (Hamilton & Sandelowski, 2004). During this early phase of developing my program of research, I was open to participant discussions and input into the incorporation of interview questions related to God as a source of social support, which led me to put aside my own bias that only mortal beings were sources of social support.

Member checking. This is another strategy frequently requested among journal reviewers necessary to enhance rigor in qualitative research. A frequent expectation of member checking to enhance rigor is for interviewers to return to participants for verification of the accuracy of either transcribed interviews or the interpretations of those interviews (Creswell, 1994). As a strategy to enhance rigor, member checking using this expectation assumes that individual memory and meanings ascribed to an experience are constant. Member checking post-interview also assumes that participants are willing to recall or engage in subsequent interpretive discussions of an experience (Sandelowski, 2008). However, the recall of a stressful life event for the purpose of interpretive validation might be burdensome to participants. In research to explore the uses of religious songs, participants were relieved to be able to talk about issues in a "safe" nonjudgmental context (Hamilton et al., 2013b, 2016). Participants who are older and living in rural areas may have had fewer opportunities for a formal education (Behringer & Krishnan, 2011). As a result, these participants may find telling their stories enjoyable, but have no interest in engaging in discussions related to interpretive meanings with researchers. Rather, validation of emerging findings as a form of member checking might be through probing for clarity of a thought or idea during the actual interview. Member checking might also be conducted using a grounded theory approach (Birt et al., 2016). For example, the interviewer might validate interpretations of experiences in subsequent interviews with participants. Probing for clarity and interpretive validation during an actual interview requires a level of skill and experience that may not be realistic in the conduct of qualitative research with underrepresented populations. When needed, I conduct a form of member checking with members of the target population who are also members of my research team.

Investigator triangulation and inter-coder reliability. Other strategies to enhance validity include using multiple methods, sources of data, investigators, or theories to confirm emerging findings (Carter et al., 2014; Merriam & Tisdel, 2016). In comparison to inter-coder reliability, I found investigator triangulation more useful in the development of categories in a previous qualitative descriptive study to understand the ways religious songs are used in response to stressful life events (Hamilton et al., 2013b). In this qualitative study, two members of the research team independently read transcripts of the interviews to clarify and to come to an agreement on definitions of emerging themes (Merriam & Tisdel, 2016; Patton, 1990). We learned that higher levels of agreement were dependent on clear, concise definitions for the emerging themes which required several meetings.

Journal reviewers may request that inter-coder reliability be used to quantify the percent in agreement. In one of our research projects, a second collaborator (of a different age, gender, and geographical region) was requested to engage in a series of face-to-face meetings to discuss categories of emerging themes until there was a consensus on the categories and their definitions. An initial meeting between myself and the collaborator resulted in a relatively low (<60%) percent agreement. During this second meeting, we determined that adding the perspective of time (i.e., whether participants referred to past, present, or future time) and person (i.e., God, self, or others) brought clarity to the definitions. In a third and final meeting, we conducted inter-coder reliability for a more robust evaluation of consistency in coding (Hamilton et al., 2013a, 2013b). Using an additional random sample of 20% of participants, Cohen's Kappa was calculated using SPSS v. 24 and deemed satisfactory (Burla et al., 2008). Other qualitative analysis programs are also useful for this process.

The contribution of inter-coder reliability to rigor is controversial and frequently applied to qualitative research indiscriminately (Morse, 2018). Moreover, while the process of inter-coder reliability is likely to contribute to clarity and simplify the codebook, the richness of the data might be lost in the iterations between coders (Morse, 2018).

Audit trail. I close this chapter on rigor with a discussion on the necessity of an audit trail. Years ago, scholars believed the audit trail was necessary in order for other researchers to replicate your study. The current stated purpose of audit trail is to have a record of the research process from the beginning with the research question, to the end with the interpretation of findings. This audit trail is to ensure that the process is transparent, allowing external reviewers to assess the trustworthiness of the project. External reviewers will judge the trustworthiness of the project through information on the research team, sampling strategies, data collection, data analysis, and conclusions drawn. I have also argued that qualitative research cannot be replicated, but it can be convincing to others that the data was obtained using rigor throughout the process.

I would also like to point out that I am frequently asked to review proposals and manuscripts using qualitative methods. Many of these proposals and manuscripts read like a textbook. As if the composer lifted the language right out of the textbook to argue that a thing was done. When I was a beginner in qualitative research, I read qualitative texts through and through and used all the language I learned from reading those texts. I purported to use axial coding and selective coding, inductive and deductive reasoning, etc. Thankfully, my mentor insisted that I tell the story of the methods section in a language that described what I had done. This continues to be my practice. To tell the reader exactly, using my own words what I did, using qualitative jargon at a minimum.

Conclusion

In this chapter, I discussed strategies that are generally accepted and promoted as standards for claiming rigor or quality in qualitative research (Morse, 2015). Of those strategies, the most critical to generating "data rich" findings are those that enable participants to tell their stories and hence be understood. I cannot overstate the value of spending quality time with participants to gain entry into their personal space. This requires respect for customs and traditions important within the community. The qualitative research projects used as exemplars in this book are similar to other studies conducted among participants in underrepresented communities. The researcher should understand that data collection in these communities is an extremely time-intensive process (Fryer et al., 2016). The added time often includes travel to isolated communities and communication with leaders why their stories are needed and how they will be used to help others with similar issues. Time to gain trust is also likely very dependent on disclosure of any ties the interviewer has to the community. Close or extended family linkages that permit potential participants to evaluate the character and trustworthiness of the interviewer might enhance trusting relationships. Gaining trust is also applicable and necessary even when the interviewer is from a similar background, culture, or racial/ethnic group (Fryer et al., 2016).

Findings that are "data rich" should also capture the heterogeneity among rural community-dwelling participants. Although African Americans share a cultural history, their beliefs, values, and attitudes toward health and health care are individually shaped by age, gender, educational level, religious affiliation, and geographical location. African Americans may live in small communities with their own unique culture with little to no experience participating in research studies (McGarvey et al., 2011). The lack of participation in research among this population may also be the result of not being asked to participate in research, rather than negative experiences with researchers and healthcare systems (Holzer et al., 2014).

Additional strategies appropriate and useful to enhance rigor focused on those that minimized researcher bias, promoted conceptual clarity, and ensured that conclusions are based solely on findings. This was best achieved with a diverse research team (i.e., race, age, gender, educational levels) that also included a member of the target population who provided input into the study design and interpretation of findings. In the analysis of findings and reporting of results, those negative cases or that single quote that didn't seem to fit were not excluded but rather a consideration for further exploration in future studies.

Increasingly, journal reviewers are requesting information on member checking and inter-coder reliability. Member checking done with participants in remote communities where access to participants is time-intensive and educational levels are low might require a deviation from the norm of returning the participants for their validation. Validation of findings and their interpretation might include member checking during the process of data collection or follow-up focus groups with other members of the target population (Kruger et al., 2012).

Finally, inter-coder reliability may be a useful strategy to enhance rigor when more than one coder is involved in qualitative content analysis (Burla et al., 2008). When sample sizes are small and the PI has the responsibility for recruiting, interviewing, and analyzing the data, inter-coder reliability with a collaborator is useful to enhance rigor with the interpretive process. In small qualitative studies, collaborators are useful in providing intersubjective interpretation through agreement with themes and definitions of themes that were initially generated by one coder (Burla et al., 2008). While the work of achieving agreement may enhance clarity, this process may downplay the richness and creativity of the findings, and invalidates the interpretative aim of qualitative research (Morse, 2018).

References

Behringer, B. and K. Krishnan. (2011). "Understanding the role of religion in cancer care in Appalachia." *South Med J* **104**(4): 295–296.

Birt, L., S. Scott, D. Cavers, C. Campbell and F. Walter. (2016). "Member checking: A tool to enhance trustworthiness or merely a nod to validation?" *Qual Health Res* **26**(13): 1802–1811.

Bowers, B., N. Jacobson and A. Krupp. (2017). "Can lay community advisors improve the clarity of research participant recruitment materials and increase the likelihood of participation?" *Res Nurs Health* **40**(1): 63–69.

Burla, L., B. Knierim, J. Barth, K. Liewald, M. Duetz and T. Abel. (2008). "From text to codings: Intercoder reliability assessment in qualitative content analysis." *Nurs Res* **57**(2): 113–117.

Buseh, A. G., P. E. Stevens, S. Millon-Underwood, S. T. Kelber and L. Townsend. (2017). "Embracing an "African Ethos" to facilitate African immigrants participation in medical genetics and genomics research." *Nurs Outlook* **65**(1): 9–17.

Carminati, L. (2018). "Generalizability in qualitative research: A tale of two traditions." *Qual Health Res* **28**(13): 2094–2101.

Carter, N., D. Bryant-Lukosius, A. DiCenso, J. Blythe and A. J. Neville. (2014). "The use of triangulation in qualitative research." *Oncol Nurs Forum* **41**(5): 545–547.

Corbie-Smith, G., M. R. Isler, M. S. Miles and B. Banks. (2012). "Community-based HIV clinical trials: An integrated approach in underserved, rural, minority communities." *Prog Community Health Partnersh* **6**(2): 121–129.

Coyne, C. A., C. Demian-Popescu and D. Friend. (2006). "Social and cultural factors influencing health in southern West Virginia: A qualitative study." *Prev Chronic Dis* **3**(4): A124.

Creswell, J. W. (1994). *Research Design: Qualitative & Quantitative Approaches*. Thousand Oaks, CA, Sage.

Dale, S. K., T. Grimes, L. Miller, A. Ursillo and M. L. Drainoni. (2017). "In our stories": The perspectives of women living with HIV on an evidence-based group intervention." *J Health Psychol* **22**(8): 1035–1045.

Easterling, L. W. (2014). "Spiritual care with Appalachians: Beyond stereotypes." *J Pastoral Care Counsel* **68**(1–2): 5.

Fryer, C. S., S. R. Passmore, R. C. Maietta, J. Petruzzelli, E. Casper, N. A. Brown, J. Butler, 3rd, M. A. Garza, S. B. Thomas and S. C. Quinn (2016). "The symbolic value and limitations of racial concordance in minority research engagement." *Qual Health Res* **26**(6): 830–841.

Gamble, V. N. (2014). "The immortal life of Henrietta lacks reconsidered." *Hastings Cent Rep* **44**(1): 1p following 48.

Garner, S. L. and M. A. Faucher. (2014). "Perceived challenges and supports experienced by the family caregiver of the older adult: A photovoice study." *J Community Health Nurs* **31**(2): 63–74.

Guba, E. G. and Y. S. Lincoln (1994). Competing Paradigms in Qualitative Research. *Handbook of Qualitative Research*. N. K. Denzin and Y. S. Lincoln. Thousand Oaks, CA, Sage: 105–117.

Hamilton, J. B., N. C. Best, J. S. Wells and V. C. Worthy (2018). "Making sense of loss through spirituality: Perspectives of African American family members who have experienced the death of a close family member to cancer." *Palliat Support Care*: **16**(6): 662–668.

Hamilton, J. B., A. D. Moore, K. A. Johnson and H. G. Koenig. (2013a). "Reading the Bible for guidance, comfort, and strength during stressful life events." *Nurs Res* **62**(3): 178–184.

Hamilton, J. B. and M. Sandelowski. (2004). "Types of social support among African American cancer patients." *Oncol Nurs Forum* **31**(4): 792–800.

Hamilton, J. B., M. Sandelowski, A. D. Moore, M. Agarwal and H. G. Koenig. (2013b). "You need a song to bring you through": The use of religious songs to manage stressful life events." *Gerontologist* **53**(1): 26–38.

Hamilton, J. B., J. M. Stewart, K. Thompson, C. Alvarez, N. C. Best, K. Amoah and I. B. Carlton-LaNey. (2017). "Younger African American Adults' use of religious songs to manage stressful life events." *J Relig Health* **56**(1): 329–344.

Hamilton, J. B., V. C. Worthy, M. J. Kurtz, J. Cudjoe and P. A. Johnstone. (2016). "Using religious songs as an integrative and complementary therapy for the management of psychological symptoms among African American cancer survivors." *Cancer Nurs* **56**(1): 329–344.

Haynes-Maslow, L., P. Godley, L. Dimartino, B. White, J. Odom, A. Richmond and W. Carpenter. (2014). "African American women's perceptions of cancer clinical trials." *Cancer Med* **3**(5): 1430–1439.

Holliday, C. E., M. Wynne, J. Katz, C. Ford and C. Barbosa-Leiker (2018). "A CBPR approach to finding community strengths and challenges to prevent youth suicide and substance abuse." *J Transcult Nurs* **29**(1): 64–73.

Holzer, J. K., L. Ellis and M. W. Merritt. (2014). "Why we need community engagement in medical research." *J Investig Med* **62**(6): 851–855.

Kruger, T. M., M. Swanson, R. E. Davis, S. Wright, K. Dollarhide and N. E. Schoenberg. (2012). "Formative research conducted in rural Appalachia to inform a community physical activity intervention." *Am J Health Promot* **26**(3): 143–151.

Lazarus, R. S. and S. Folkman. (1984). *Stress, Appraisal, and Coping*. New York, Springer Publishing Company.

LeCompte, M. D. and J. J. Schensul. (1999). *Designing and Conducting Ethnographic Research*. Walnut Creek, CA, AltaMira Press.

Lee, H., P. Kiang, M. Kim, S. Semino-Asaro, M. E. Colten, S. S. Tang, P. Chea, S. Peou and D. C. Grigg-Saito. (2015). "Using qualitative methods to develop a contextually tailored instrument: Lessons learned." *Asia Pac J Oncol Nurs* **2**(3): 192–202.

Maxwell, J. A. (2013). *Qualitative Research Design: An Interactive Approach*. Thousand Oaks, CA, Sage Publications, Inc.

McGarvey, E. L., M. Leon-Verdin, L. F. Killos, T. Guterbock and W. F. Cohn. (2011). "Health disparities between Appalachian and non-Appalachian counties in Virginia USA." *J Community Health* **36**(3): 348–356.

Merriam, S. B. and E. J. Tisdel. (2016). *Qualitative Research: A Guide to Design and Implementation*. San Francisco, CA, Jossey-Bass.

Morse, J. (2018). Reframing Rigor in Qualitative Inquiry. *The Sage Handbook of Qualitative Research*. N. K. Denzin and Y. S. Lincoln. Thousand Oaks, CA, Sage Publications: 796–817.

Morse, J. M. (2015). "Critical analysis of strategies for determining rigor in qualitative inquiry." *Qual Health Res* **25**(9): 1212–1222.

Patton, M. Q. (1990). *Qualitative Evaluation and Research Methods*. Newbury Park, CA, Sage.

Ponterotto, J. G. (2010). "Qualitative research in multicultural psychology: Philosophical underpinnings, popular approaches, and ethical considerations." *Cultur Divers Ethnic Minor Psychol* **16**(4): 581–589.

Presley, C. (2013). "Cultural awareness: Enhancing clinical experiences in rural Appalachia." *Nurse Educ* **38**(5): 223–226.

Sandelowski, M. (2008). Member Check. *The SAGE Encyclopedia of Qualitative Research Methods*. L. Given. Thousand Oaks, CA, Sage: 501–502.

Schwandt, T. A. (2000). Three Epistemological Studies for Qualitative Inquiry: Interpretivism, Hermeneutics, and Social Constructionism. *Handbook of Qualitative Research*. N. K. Denzin and Y. S. Lincoln (Eds.). Thousand Oaks, CA, Sage Publishers: 189–213.

Stewart, J. M. (2015). "A multi-level approach for promoting HIV testing within African American church settings." *AIDS Patient Care STDS* **29**(2): 69–76.

White, R. M. (2003). "The Tuskegee syphilis study and consent." *Ann Emerg Med* **42**(3): 430–431; author reply 431.

9 Coding Schemes

In this chapter, I discuss the process of coding and provide examples from my research on topics that include *Data Management* (labeling and storing interview data, managing transcripts), *Identifying Themes and Categories* (coding strategies to generate tentative theory and to identify themes and categories). The exemplar coding strategies are from my research using grounded theory techniques to explore social support experiences among African American cancer survivors. Discussions on *Data Management* and *Identifying Themes and Categories* include text, diagrams, and tables to illustrate how I developed a coding style.

Data Management

Labeling and storing qualitative data. Immediately after completing the interview or focus group, I download the data into a password-protected computer or password protected and encrypted external hard drive (our University Informational Technology personnel assists with encryption). All interviews are downloaded to a numbered file. I may use a number that represents the participant number and year of study or a number where I assign the study a number, then participant number, and year of the study. So, if the study number is 05, participant number is 01, and study year is 2025, the file of participant number 01 would be 05-01-2025. I always have a backup copy of audio-recorded interviews. Audio files are then uploaded to a secure university one drive folder and shared with the transcriptionist. The transcriptionist is an individual I have worked with for several years. She is familiar with the verbal expressions of my target population who frequently have low levels of education and may use jargon not easily understood or picked up by electronic transcription devices.

Managing transcriptions. The transcriptionist uses verbatim transcription to capture authentic dialogue, word-for-word, in an effort to capture any emotions or emphasis used during the conversation or interview. Using any confidentiality guidelines provided by the investigator, she eliminates any identifiers from the transcripts. This can be achieved by either redacting the identifiable information or assigning a pseudonym. Generally, pseudonyms are provided by the researcher, or the transcriptionist uses a random name generator to assign one. Additionally, for the actual respondent in the interview, the transcriptionist labels the voices of the participants as respondent 1, or participant 1, etc. If any issues are encountered with audibility, [brackets] are used to indicate a part of the interview was left out because it was inaudible. Alternatively, when the transcriptionist has a reasonable guess of a word or a phrase, that phrase will be typed and placed in [brackets], letting the researcher know the wording of this text needs to be confirmed. If a respondent

DOI: 10.4324/9781003598916-9

Table 9.1 Example Transcript

HAMILTON:	Alright, so this is week three and this is your last week of looking at videos.
033-2022:	Okay.
HAMILTON:	And then we have one more time to do that questionnaire thing again. And we can do that later in the week.
033-2022:	Okay.
HAMILTON:	Whenever you get ready.
033-2022:	I'm ready now.
HAMILTON:	Okay, so, now for today though, it's about those five videos.
033-2022:	Mmhm?
HAMILTON:	I really cared a lot about what happened to the characters. Not at all, a little, somewhat, a lot, quite a bit.
033-2022:	Quite a bit.
033-2022_CL:	Yes. Quite a bit. Mmhm.?
HAMILTON:	Events in the stories could happen in my community.
033-2022_CL:	Yes, ma'am. They do and have. Yes, ma'am.
HAMILTON:	I found the stories enjoyable.
033-2022_CL:	Mmmm.
HAMILTON:	Did you enjoy them? Did you enjoy them?
033-2022_CL:	Well (stammers), I related to them. I mean, I don't know if I enjoyed them, but they are what they are. (Laughs).
HAMILTON:	Oh okay. So, you're thinking enjoy watching people suffering or did you enjoy just watching?
033-2022_CL:	I mean I, I like hearing about our stories. I love to hear about us surviving.

displays any audible emotions, or changes tone or volume—for example, starts to whisper or yell—she will add that note, using parentheses (laughing), (starts to sob), (yells), (emphasizes), (Stammers)... This is important to help demonstrate context or emotions or to help the reviewer get a sense of not only what is said but how it is said. Also, if a person starts to say something and then changes their conversation mid-sentence, three dots (...) are used to indicate that an expressed thought was incomplete. During a focus group, should multiple people speak over each other (talk at the same time), the transcriptionist will try to separate those voices. If this is not possible, the transcriptionist will attempt to capture as much of what was said as possible and then indicate [overlapping talk] to the researcher these are parts of the conversation that couldn't be captured. Table 9.1 is an exemplar of a transcribed interview. Notice how the transcriptionist separates the interview questions from the participant responses. Also the interviewer or PI name is used but the participant is identified only by initials and number.

Demographics. In my early years of learning to code, I created a summary demographic table for each participant (Hamilton, 2001). The table below captured essential information including date of interview, demographic characteristics (situational and clinical). I was able to refer back to this summary during analysis and also during manuscript writing. In the table following, I constructed an elaborate demographic display with demographic characteristics as well as categories for each participant. As I became more experienced, I kept this information in a notebook, and the information in the

Table 9.2 Example of Summary Demographics

Date of interview	*July 22, 1998*
Age	63 years
Date of diagnosis	1994
Date ended participation in primary study	1/95
Cancer stage	Staging not available
Cancer treatment	Surgery
Residence	Wilson, NC
Years education	16 years, 2 associate degrees
Employment status	Retired
Employment history	Worked previously in a furniture store
Marital status	Married
Number children	2 adult children, daughters
Persons Living in Home	Lives in house with wife, daughter and granddaughter
Proximity to Other Family Members	Other family members
Co-Morbidities	None
Church Membership	Attends church, teaches new members class
Years Residing in Current Community	Lived in community most of adult life
Primary Study Treatment Cell	Treatment Direct

demographic display was entered into a statistical quantitative program. See examples in Tables 9.2 and 9.3.

Table 9.4, I illustrate the use of fictitious names assigned to participants prior to analysis. These fictious names are useful with efforts to maintain anonymity, but also to visualize the participant as a person during analysis. The names are of favorite authors or childhood mentors.

Generating Tentative Theory, Themes, and Categories

In this next section, I describe in detail the ways in which I manually coded interview data using grounded theory techniques (Hamilton, 2001). As previously noted, during my novice years, I played around with a ton of tables until I eventually landed on my own unique style of coding. These tables are exemplars from my dissertation research and included for illustration purposes.

Coding with Grounded Theory

In this first section on coding with Grounded Theory, I describe the ways in which I coded and analyzed data from the in-person interviews with 15 African American women with breast cancer and 13 African American men with prostate cancer to understand their experiences with social support (Hamilton, 2001). The data used to code and analyze the *Theorizing Social Support* project were typed transcripts of the audiotapes, study field notes, and demographic data. Interviews were typed verbatim and checked for accuracy. These typed transcriptions as raw data were initially entered into the computer as individual cases using

Table 9.3 Example Demographic Display

Case	*Age*	*Marital status*	*Education*	*Employment*	*Residence*	*Family*	*Child in home*	*Years in neighborhood*	*Group member*	*Family in town*	*Advice/ info*	*Distract*	*Encour*	*God*	*Instru*	*Presence*	*Protect*
1	52	Divorced	12	Medical Leave	Urban	Yes	No	Since adult	No	Yes	Yes	Yes	Yes	Yes	Yes	Yes	Yes
2	65	Single	10	Retired	Urban	Yes	No	Since adult	Yes	Yes	Yes	Yes	Yes	Yes	Yes	Yes	Yes
3	54	Widowed	10	Medical Leave	Urban	Yes	No	Since adult	No	Yes	Yes	Yes	Yes	Yes	Yes	Yes	Yes
4	80	Widowed	10	Retired	Urban	No	No	Since adult	No	Yes	Yes	No	Yes	Yes	Yes	Yes	No
5	52	Single	12	Full time	Urban	Yes	Yes	Recent	No	No	Yes	Yes	Yes	Yes	Yes		Yes
6	58	Married	12	Unemployed	Urban	Yes	No	Since adult	Yes	Yes	Yes	Yes	Yes	Yes	Yes	Yes	Yes
7	66	Married	8	Retired	Urban	Yes	No	Since adult	No	Yes	Yes	Yes	No	Yes	Yes	Yes	Yes
8	52	Married	12	Medical Leave	Rural	Yes	Yes	Since adult	Yes	Yes	Yes	No	Yes	No	Yes	Yes	No
9	58	Married	12	Medical Leave	Urban	Yes	No	Since adult	No	No	Yes	Yes	Yes	Yes	Yes	Yes	Yes
10	87	Widowed	16	Retired	Urban	No	No	Since adult	Yes	Yes	No	Yes	Yes	Yes	Yes	Yes	Yes
11	69	Separated	16	Retired	Urban	Yes	No	Since adult	Yes	Yes	Yes	Yes	Yes	Yes	Yes	Yes	Yes
12	58	Married	19	Retired	Urban	Yes	No	Since adult	Yes	Yes	Yes	Yes	Yes	Yes	Yes	Yes	Yes
13	61	Widowed	18	Retired	Urban	Yes	No	Since adult	Yes	Yes	Yes	Yes	Yes	Yes	Yes	Yes	Yes
14	42	Married	16	Full time	Rural	Yes	Yes	Since adult	No	Yes	Yes	Yes	Yes	Yes	Yes	Yes	Yes
15	45	Married	18	Full time	Urban	Yes	No	Since adult	yes	No	Yes	Yes	Yes	Yes	Yes	Yes	Yes

Table 9.4 Example Table for Fictious Names

Fictious names women		*Fictious names men*	
C01	Ms. Angelo	AA01	Mr. Malcom
C02	Ms. White	AA02	Mr. Neighbors
C03	Ms. Collins	AA03	Mr. Gaines
C04	Ms. Jones	AA04	Mr. Dressler
C05	Ms. Cooper	AA05	Mr. Ellison
C06	Ms. Farmer	AA06	Mr. Franklin
C07	Ms. Sojourner	AA07	Mr. Gutman
C08	Ms. Brent	AA08	Mr. Higginbotham
C09	Ms. McAdoo	AA09	Mr. Gates
C10	Ms. Hurston	AA10	Mr. Logan
C11	Ms. Hine	AA11	Mr. Hooks
C12	Ms. Lerner	AA12	Mr. West
C13	Ms. Morrison	AA13	Mr. Sherrill
C14	Ms. Naylor		
C15	Ms. Painter		

the qualitative data analysis software Non-numerical Unstructured Data Indexing Searching and Theorizing (QSR NUDIST 4.0 for Windows). I also entered process notes that I made during the interview in which I recorded some behavioral observations, the presence of other persons in the home, aspects of the neighborhood, and any emotions such as crying, expressed during the interview. I eventually adopted a manual process that permitted greater flexibility with coding data from participants who consistently varied constantly on the language used to describe their social support experiences. Recorded observations were useful when describing participants in the findings of oral and written presentations.

I selected the grounded theory approach for my dissertation since the goal was to understand social support from the African American cancer survivor perspective. I was sensitized by existing research that focused on white and middle-class populations but very little research had been conducted on African Americans. I especially appreciated the grounded theory approach of beginning the interview with a limited number of semi-structured questions that permitted the participant to describe their experiences in their own words. Probing followed the participant comments rather than a list of preconceived questions based on what was known in the literature. I also appreciated that the grounded theory approach to data analysis was guided by a constant comparative method (Strauss & Corbin, 1998). Constant comparison of the data is the process of continually asking questions and making comparisons of the data. These comparisons assisted with the identification of patterns or variations in the data both within each interview and across interviews.

I initially began to analyze each transcribed interview by looking for the language used to describe social support experiences. I created a table with columns of this language and very brief quotes from participants. I also compared interviews according to groups along the key variables selected (gender, education, income, proximity to family, and geographical location). For example, I compared transcribed interviews (cases) of women to women; unmarried women to married women; more educated women with less educated women; women in rural areas to women in urban areas; and women living alone to women living

Table 9.5 Example Case by Case Coding

Initial Case by Case Coding

Initially started data analysis examining individual cases of women to identify uniqueness of each case.

I read each case through initially to pull out demographics about the case that were in addition to those collected during the interview. This information seemed to have an effect on either the person providing the support or the type of support provided. For example, during the analysis of C001, the fact that the participant had lived in her neighborhood seemed to determine the number or persons in her network and also the type of support available to her. Also type and/or place of employment seemed to affect the participants' level of anxiety about their cancer experience and the type of support they felt they needed. For example, C001 had worked in a hospital and seemed to be less nervous about her treatment because she "knew the nurses that worked there." And, because she was an employee, the nurses allowed family members to be with her during times that were restricted to other patients.

A third demographic factor that seemed to influence the numbers of network members and the type of support provided by those members was whether or not the participant was a church member or attended church.

During this interview, three additional demographic factors were added: (1) length of time in neighborhood, (2) type employment, and (3) church membership or attendance.

After I identified demographic factors that seemed to influence the participants' social support experiences, I started line-by-line coding to identify social network members and the type of support provided. I also identified persons talked to about cancer and other problems and persons not talked to. I also put into a category all those things the participant did to make herself feel better during her experience with cancer.

Initial phrases, sentences were sorted into categories of help receiving and giving for C001. I also began the process of giving these categories initial labels. These were family and friends who indicated they were there for me; family and friends called me and came by to visit; family and/ or friends came by to sit with me; family and friends sent me cards, flowers, and they collected money for me. Encouraging words from others seen as positive were "you don't look sick," you look good. This participant stated throughout the interview that she didn't get that sick (I am not sure what that meant).

with a spouse or other family member. These same comparisons were also made with the men. Finally, the cases of men were compared to the cases of women. Table 9.5 is an exemplar of initial case by case coding of phenomena of interest (social support). Notice in the example below my initial thinking and summary of social network members and the types of support exchanged in the case of participant number C001.

After this initial review of cases along key variables, I returned to look at each individual interview as a case to get to know the "whole person." Each individual case was examined to determine an initial typology of social support experiences unique to each case. I also explored similarities and differences with this emerging typology in each individual case and also among groups according to key variables mentioned previously. If my goal had been to generate tentative theory, I would have explored each individual case for antecedents and consequences to the social support experience. In other words, I would have explored the factors that influenced the participant's experiences with social support and also the outcomes from those social support experiences. However, for the purpose of generating a typology of social support, each individual interview was examined to determine those participants' experiences with social support but also what factors influence those person's experiences and to determine the outcomes of those experiences. I also compared those experiences to those of other participants to determine which experiences were similar and which were different.

Once individual cases were summarized, I proceeded with the coding scheme as outlined in Strauss and Corbin (1998). According to Strauss & Corbin, there are three types of coding used to develop theory that is grounded in data: Open, Axial, and Selective coding. Open coding is the process of initially generating categories and exploring relationships among those categories. During open coding, I analyzed each line, sentence and paragraph of text to identify words or phrases associated with events or actions used to express experiences of social support (Strauss & Corbin, 1998). For example, any sentences or phrases with the words "helped me with" or "they came to do" or "went with me" were sorted into categories of social support. Manual coding was conducted to sort similar concepts together and to place these concepts into a table with columns to capture concepts related to social support.

Axial coding was done to reconstruct the data into related categories and subcategories of concepts to explain the phenomenon of social support as expressed in these interviews. Again, had the goal been tentative theory, Axial coding would have been the process of examining the set of circumstances in which the phenomenon was rooted, individual or group responses to those circumstances, and the consequences or outcomes that occurred as a result of the phenomenon (Strauss & Corbin, 1998). According to the larger body of social support literature, some circumstances or issues that have influenced social support experiences have been the need to talk about illness or the need to know more about a physical symptom. Individual responses to those circumstances or issues have been to talk to family members and friends about their illness-related concerns. When the issue has been a concern about a physical symptom, some individual responses have been to seek out professional advice or assistance. Finally, a consequence or outcome from a social support experience has been a reduction in anxiety, depression, or strength to endure cancer treatments. For my study to generate a typology of social support, I used axial coding to make relational statements among types of social support used in response to the stress of a cancer diagnosis. For example, the end goal was to construct a table of an expanded conceptualization of emotional support, instrumental support, and informational support. This axial coding resulted in 11 categories of types of social support. As you will see in Table 9.6, I began coding the interview data according to different types of social support, the antecedents, context, intervening conditions, actions/interactions, and consequences. Antecedents lead up to the type of social support given or received. Context was the situation under which the social support was given or received. Intervening conditions influenced the receipt of the type of social support. Actions/interactions were specific (subcategories) of a type of social support. Lastly, consequences were the patient's outcome from the social support given or received.

Selective coding was the process of integrating and refining categories to form a larger theoretical scheme (typology) or theory of social support (Strauss & Corbin, 1998). In this *Theorizing Social Support* project, selective coding allowed me to revise and refine the initial categories of social support. During this phase of coding, I focused on two major activities: (1) refining definitions of concepts and relational statements (typology) into the final product and (2) integration of concepts into relational statements to explain the transactional nature of social support for African American cancer patients. Specifically for this project, I used constant comparison to revise, refine, and fill in gaps of emerging categories of social support and to explore patterns of reciprocity that occurred during supportive interactions among African American cancer patients.

In Table 9.7, I illustrate my initial effort to refine a typology of social support. Using constant comparison, I filled in poorly developed categories, trimmed excess data, and reduced the initial typology of social support. I identified gaps in the emerging typology

Table 9.6 Example Coding for Tentative Theory

Type of social support	*Antecedent conditions*	*Context*	*Intervening conditions*	*Actions/Interactions*	*Consequences/Outcomes*
Exchanging advice and information	Being told of cancer diagnosis Needing to select a physician Needing to validate information from MD Needing to make treatment decision Needing to validate treatment decision Wanting information about diagnosis and treatment Needing help to manage side effects of cancer treatments Wanting to help others be screened Wanting to help others seek treatment Wanting to help others through treatment and side effects Wanting to be an example to others	During initial phases of diagnosis and during treatment During later phases of cancer diagnosis, after recovery from treatment	Persons providing advice and information more accepted from healthcare professional or person with similar experience Physician with similar religious faith and from similar ethnic background more trustworthy Fear of revealing diagnosis of cancer to others Fear of stigma or negative comments from others Inaccurate information Conflicting information Mistrust of Healthcare System and Physicians (provider intent) History of consulting with informal network members prior to seeking help from formal healthcare professionals Access to family members, friends with healthcare experience.	Talking to others who are knowledgeable of the healthcare system Listening to stories about others with similar experiences Reading pamphlets containing cancer-related information Looking at TV programs Getting questions answered	Worries decreased Anxiety levels decreased Proceed with treatment Prepared/informed about what to expect during treatment Comparisons with others let them know whether they were progressing or not, let them know they were not the only ones with this illness Helps to know others have gone through this and survived Good feelings about treatment decision Able to manage side effects from treatment Able to get questions answered The receipt of inaccurate information caused anger and mistrust Felt good to help someone else by sharing their experiences Felt good being able to teach others about the importance of being screened Too much advice from friends was confusing

(*Continued*)

Table 9.6 (Continued)

Type of social support	*Antecedent conditions*	*Context*	*Intervening conditions*	*Actions/Interactions*	*Consequences/Outcomes*
Made to feel needed	Needing to maintain usual social roles with families and church Needing to feel important to others Needing to feel useful	During initial phases of diagnosis and treatment Responsible for the care of an elderly relative Responsible for the care of a younger child or grandchild	Not being able to manage side effects Worries about appearance (loss of hair, leaking urine, breast prosthesis)	Church members held positions, delayed activities within the church Family members performed the work, family roles for participant, i.e. Being told by others they are missed	When you feel needed, it makes you want to fight to get better Felt good to know that you are needed by others Keeps participants from thinking or worrying about themselves and their problems Give participants something to live for
Presence	Needing treatment for cancer Not being able to get out, being confined to hospital or home	During treatment	Being active in church and community groups may facilitate the amounts Living in neighborhoods for a long time Not having to ask Expectations for visiting and calling depend on perspective of participant (?daughters expected to be physically present, frequency of calls, visits based on perspective of participant. Maybe it depends on previous relationship, see AA01, AA08, gender roles)	Coming by to visit on a regular basis Calling on a regular basis Sitting with participant Doing nothing, others are just there Reassuring words from others that they would always be there, are accepting of the participants condition Having family move back home to be with them Being available should anything be needed	Helps to get through it [the treatment]. Gives participants the strength to get through the treatments Communicates that others are willing to share the burden Some people who come or curious, not sincere Relationships with others maintained

(*Continued*)

Table 9.6 (Continued)

Type of social support	*Antecedent conditions*	*Context*	*Intervening conditions*	*Actions/Interactions*	*Consequences/Outcomes*
Avoidance behaviors	Feeling that no one will understand their problems Not wanting to burden others with problems Fearing negative comments	During the initial phases, i.e., diagnosis, treatment	Belief that nothing can help, can be done Fear of stigma Myths of side effects, survival rates of cancer Fear of loosing	Staying away from others Going someplace to be alone Limited or no visiting others	Limited amounts or no support received from others Limited or no opportunities to share experiences with others, support others
Distracting Activities	Worrying about outcome of cancer diagnosis Sitting around the house, not being able to get out to do usual activities, bored Feeling depressed	During the treatment and after recovery	History of joking about other stressful life events Coping style when worrying	Engaging in social activities with others Staying busy doing things Attempts to make light of the situation Attempts to not focus on the negatives of the situation	Helps take your mind off your worries if you're focused on something else Keeps you going Helpful to stay busy
Encouraging words	Diagnosis of cancer Being told by MD some form of cancer treatment needed	During diagnosis, treatment, recovery and beyond	Concern about appearances Perceived intent of comments	Telling others how good they look Validating the participants decision to have treatment Telling others to be screened for cancer	Good feelings about treatment decision Good feelings about appearance Side effects of cancer treatment are minimized Able to get others to get screened or treated for cancer Given strength to continue treatments Not helpful if perceived as not sincere Intimate relationships maintained

(*Continued*)

Table 9.6 (Continued)

Type of social support	*Antecedent conditions*	*Context*	*Intervening conditions*	*Actions/Interactions*	*Consequences/Outcomes*
Help from God	Worries about problems Worries about diagnosis of cancer Being sick from cancer treatments Feeling depressed Needing to talk to someone when no one else is there or will understand	During initial phases, treatment, recovery, and beyond	Faith in an all powerful, protective God Belief that God is available all the time Past experiences with God, religion	Praying (turning troubles over to God) Reading the Bible Meditating Prayer groups Religious TV programs	Calming feeling Worries removed Feelings of being prepared for any outcome Feeling of not being alone Belief that God has healed the cancer Prayer is like a medication Survived treatment Illness controlled Given strength to continue usual activities
Protecting/ monitoring	Not wanting to worry others or be a burden to others Family members, friends wanting to monitor progress to treatment	During initial phases of diagnosing, treatment	Not accepting support from others Wanting to do for self Valuing being independent, self-reliant	Checking on the participants response to treatment, progress Family members, friends trying to protect participant from further harm (returning to usual activities too soon, doing too much work, going too much, following prescribed treatments, diet)	Too much protecting from family is perceived as harmful

(*Continued*)

Table 9.6 (Continued)

Type of social support	*Antecedent conditions*	*Context*	*Intervening conditions*	*Actions/Interactions*	*Consequences/Outcomes*
Self-reliance (resourcefulness)	Not having others to depend on Not wanting to ask others for help Not wanting to disclose problems Not wanting to depend on others	During diagnosis, treatment, recovery, and beyond	Ability to return to usual activities Having served in roles of responsibility (See John Henryism)	Doing things to make oneself feel better Continuing to do as much for self as possible Refusal to take on sick role	Being strong helped them through this experience Helps through recovery
Sharing/offers to help	Helping others who are sick and shut in (grounded in religion)	During diagnosis, treatment phases (this type help decreases when participant is in recovery phase of illness	Disclosure to someone about cancer diagnosis Having to ask for help is a barrier Fear of rejection Fear of being a burden to others Access to financial resources	Offers to help with household chores Contributions of money Providing transportation Assisting with nursing care needs Assisting with work, family and church responsibilities	Feelings of being cared about, appreciated Not really needed but makes you feel that someone cares Calming Brightens your day Financial independence maintained
Positive thinking	Cancer Experience	During treatment, recovery, and time beyond	Wanting to make sense of cancer experience (see Sontag) Past history of losses (experience with deaths of family members) Style of coping	Not thinking about it as cancer Not talking about it much Thinking that this is just another one of life's hurdles Accepting a change in one's health Thinking things could be worse Feeling as if I am not dying Seeing oneself as not as sick as others	Acceptance of changes in one's health Able to manage worries (regain, maintain control over self)

Table 9.7 Example Typology Social Support Concepts with Revised Definitions

Category	*Definition*
Advice or information	*The receipt of advice, information, guidance through stages of diagnosis or treatment. Also includes selection of MD or treatment facility. Hearing about others experiences with cancer.* *Similar to existing category Informational Support.*
Being needed	*Helped through expressions of being needed to do something or to care for someone.*
Being there	*Verbal replies or actions of being there The giving of one's self. The readiness of others in anticipation of the need for something. Can be verbal expression, physical presence* *(See presence literature).*
Distancing/not telling	*Staying away from Situations/People perceived as negative or that may trigger negative thoughts (See Avoidance coping among AA in cancer literature) **Note(1/18/2001) Not Telling to avoid negative rumors, having people treat you differently)*
Discouraging words/comments	*Verbal expressions from others that are perceived as negative. Telling the person he or she should not have been treated for cancer. Treating the person differently as if they are dying.*
Distracting activities	*Having others help to divert or take mind off worries by not talking about the problem, engaging in activities to stay busy such as walking, shopping, getting out. Diversionary activities seen as positive by participant.* *(See Levine—black laughter, use of humor)*
Encouraging words	*Verbal expressions from others that are perceived as inspiring. Also urging the person to seek treatment or proceed with prescribed medical treatments. Includes comments about one's appearance that are perceived as positive.*
Help from God/praying	*The perception of being helped by having faith in God and prayer. Turning negative emotions over to God. Helped received directly from God (See caregiving lit, Parham & Wood, Picot, religiosity literature).*
Protecting behaviors	*Actions to guard someone from something. Also monitoring or checking on the condition of the persons' progress.*
Self-reliance	*Helped through doing things to take care of self. Read Self-Help Carrie Braden*
Sharing/offers to help	*The giving or receiving of some good or service or the offering of such. Similar to the existing category of instrumental support. Includes the act of doing something, i.e., praying for someone. Help to maintain same life, to maintain social roles, jobs*
Thoughts	*Helped through self-generated positive thinking. (see autobiography-Life is so good)*
Controlling rumors	*Telling others the facts about the diagnosis/illness to prevent negative rumors/gossip. The anticipation that rumors are minimized or prevented through telling the facts before others make erroneous conclusions.*

of social support by constantly questioning ideas presented in the narratives and tables. Questions asked of the data focused on whether this typology made sense and reflected experiences with social support versus some other concept. Filling in poorly developed categories was accomplished by either reviewing the raw data for more information or collecting additional data from other sources. Throughout the analysis phase, I returned to sources of information on the social support experiences of African Americans from historical literature, published biographies, and autobiographies. Information from this literature helped me to expand my thinking and fill in gaps on social support. Specifically, I gained an understanding of the contexts surrounding social and cultural influences impacting the Black family. This step of coding resulted in 13 categories of social support.

The third step in revising and refining this typology was to trim or drop excess data or ideas expressed in the interviews that did not relate to experiences of social support. This final step in refining theory is the process of validating the theory. Validating the theory developed in this project was accomplished by determining if the categories of social support could explain the experiences of a majority of the individual cases. In this step, it is advised to "try out" the labeling of categories with their definitions on other African Americans with cancer or community partners. In other words, the categories and definitions could be validated among African Americans who have similar cancer diagnoses and treatment experiences and to determine whether these categories are consistent with their social support experiences. In the table below, I continued to refine and collapse the typology of social support and detail the definitions for each category. In this next step, Table 9.8, I continued to refine the categories and definitions and collapsed the categories of social support to nine.

Table 9.8 Example Further Refinement of Typology of Social Support

Type of Support from Network Members			
Advice or information	*Being there*	*Distracting activities*	*Encouraging words*
The receipt of advice, information, guidance through stages of diagnosis or treatment. Also includes selection of MD or treatment facility and hearing about others similar experiences.	*Verbal replies or actions of being there The giving of one's self. The availability of others in anticipation of the need for something. Can be verbal expression, physical presence.*	*Having others help to distract or take mind off worries by not talking about the problem, engaging in activities to stay busy such as walking, shopping, getting out.*	*Verbal expressions from others that are perceived as encouraging. Also encouragement to seek treatment or proceed with prescribed medical treatments. Includes positive comments about one's appearance.*
Help from God/praying	*Helping others*	*Protecting behaviors*	*Sharing/offers to help*
The perception of being helped by having faith in God and prayer. Turning negative emotions over to God.	*The perception of helping others by sharing personal experiences. Also being able to maintain social roles of giving such as in Church or community organizations.*	*Actions to protect someone. Can be protection from having to worry, communication of information that would be upsetting.*	*The actual receipt of some good or service or the offering of such. Similar to the category of instrumental support. Includes people offering prayers.*

The intended product of this research will be a culturally relevant typology of social support for African Americans with a life-threatening illness such as cancer. Having a culturally relevant typology of social support for African Americans will serve to increase our knowledge of social support as experienced by this population. This typology, grounded in the experiences of African Americans, will also be a valuable guide to future intervention studies for this minority population.

In Table 9.9, I constructed a final typology of categories of social support with definitions. I continued to rename categories and refine definitions. This final typology of nine categories was integrated with existing categories of social support as types of emotional, instrumental, and informational support.

In addition to the tables displaying text with type categories and definitions, it may be useful to the reader to present data in numbers. For example, the table below displays the numbers of participants with quotes from each category. The categories have been rank-ordered from highest to lowest in frequency according to gender.

Table 9.9 Example Final Typology of Social Support

Social Support as Types of Emotional, Instrumental, Informational Support		
Category	*Subcategory*	*Definition*
Emotional support	Presence of others	A communication of verbal and nonverbal behaviors from network members that they are available and willing to help in whatever way needed; a form of companionship.
	Encouraging words	A verbal communication from network members the cancer patient perceives as positive, uplifting, motivating; to reassure or to encourage positive self-evaluation.
	Distracting activities	Diversionary activities provided by network members; behaviors from network members to divert the cancer patient's mind from the cancer experience and related problems or concerns.
	Protecting/monitoring	Actions or behaviors done to guard, shield someone against something. To protect from further harm.
Instrumental support	Offers of prayers	A communication from network members that they are praying for the cancer patient.
	Assistance to maintain social roles	Assistance from network members to help the cancer patient maintain social roles in their workplace, churches, or families/homes.
	Assistance to continue religious practices	Support from network members to assist the cancer patient in continuing religious practices—Holy Communion, tithing, conducting religious services outside of the church.
	Assistance to continue living in the home	Having network members move in permanently or temporarily allows the cancer patient to continue living at home.
Informational support	Advice/information	Similar to existing definitions of informational support. Includes giving and receiving advice, information, and guidance about cancer. Also includes assistance to select physician or treatment facility.

Table 9.10 Categories of Types of Social Support by Gender (N = 28)

Categories	*Women*	*Men*	*Total*
Sharing/offers to help	15	13	28
Presence of others	14	12	26
Help from God	12	12	24
Advice/information	12	11	23
Encouraging words	11	11	22
Distraction	11	9	20
Protection/monitoring	11	9	20

Table 9.11 Type of Support used by Gender (N = 65)

	Women n = 46		*Men n = 19*		
	n	*(%)*	*n*	*(%)*	X^2
Sharing/offers to help	33	71.7	7	36.8	6.92**
Presence of others	14	30.4	1	5.3	4.80*
Help from God	7	15.2	3	15.8	.00
Advice/information	6	13.0	4	21.1	.66
Encouraging words	5	10.9	1	5.3	.50
Distraction	3	6.5	6	31.6	7.08**
Protecting/monitoring	1	2.2	1	5.3	.43

* $p \leq .05$
** $p \leq .01$
Note: Participants could have used more than one type of Bible verse.

However, you may also find it helpful to display numbers according to another demographic (educational level, income, marital status, etc.), or even percentiles. In studies where sample sizes were larger than 20, I have even conducted nonparametric analysis to determine whether numerical differences among categories were statistically significant. See examples of displaying numbers for categories of social support in Tables 9.10 and 9.11.

Conclusion

In this chapter, I discussed strategies to manage data and coding for tentative theory, themes, and categories. Although generating a tentative theory using grounded theory techniques was an initial goal with my dissertation research, I switched to the identification of the typology of social support to be consistent with my future goal to develop a new measure of social support. In the next chapter, I discuss data analysis strategies used to identify and name themes and categories using *Content Analysis* and *Thematic Analysis*. I also briefly discuss quantitative analysis used to describe participants and explore group differences using Chi-square and Fisher's exact testing.

References

Hamilton, J. (2001). *Theorizing social support among African Americans with cancer*. Doctoral Dissertation, University of North Carolina.

Strauss, A. and J. Corbin. (1998). *Basics of Qualitative Research: Techniques and Procedures for Developing Grounded Theory*. Thousand Oaks, CA, Sage.

10 Qualitative Analysis Strategies

In this chapter, I discuss strategies for analysis and provide examples from my research on topics that include identifying and naming categories (subcategories) or themes (subthemes). Specifically, I primarily focus on content analysis but using hypothetical examples, I include a brief discussion on thematic analysis. I conclude this chapter with a discussion of ways I have used quantitative analysis to report participant demographics and examinations of statistical difference among frequencies of categories.

Content Analysis

Content Analysis has been my preference for the analysis of qualitative data. This strategy is flexible and permits analysis when guided by theory. It is used (or not) or when concepts are related (or not) (Hsieh & Shannon, 2005). Hsieh and Shannon (2005) describe three approaches to content analysis: (1) conventional, (2) directed, or (3) summative. Conventional content analysis is a type of analysis that identifies codes directly from text data that can be from one-on-one interviews, open-ended survey questions, focus groups, observations, or even print media. Using this approach to analysis, the data is explored to provide the reader with knowledge or understanding of the phenomena of interest and is useful whether or not the project is guided by an explicitly stated framework. In this next section, I will provide three examples of content analysis from my research with African American cancer patients.

In the first example, content analysis was conducted to analyze the narratives of 18 African American women to explore their experiences with stressors during the COVID pandemic and the way they responded to these stressors. A qualitative descriptive approach was appropriate given the goal of the study was to simply report these participants' reports of stressors encountered and their responses to these stressors. The study was not guided by an explicitly stated theory or the findings from published research. There were no preconceived categories for coding, and minimal interpretations of the coded data. A qualitative descriptive approach allowed me to pull from strategies from other approaches in order to collect the best data to answer the research question. In this toolkit, I generally draw from my research training in grounded theory to use constant comparison and maximum variation (Strauss & Corbin, 1998). If you recall, with constant comparison, I am continually asking questions and making comparisons of the data within each case and across each case. These comparisons assisted with the identification of patterns or variations in the data both within each interview and across interviews. Also given that the voice of the African American cancer survivor is limited in research, I never begin a

DOI: 10.4324/9781003598916-10

study with more than four interview questions. Fewer questions allow me to follow the conversation and probe where the participant leads. Even if the participant introduces information that I have not anticipated, I capture that content and explore with the participant their thinking of how the information is related to the purpose of the study. If there is not a fit, I still explore that topic with other participants. In some cases, this information has led to an extension of the research question or information to be coded for a separate manuscript. Bottom line, I never discard any data collected, all data are important and are reported in the findings of oral presentations and/or manuscripts.

In addition to a qualitative descriptive approach to guide the sampling and interview questions (Sandelowski, 2010), I used conventional content analysis to guide the coding scheme. Using this approach, I read the first transcript word for word and made notes of my thoughts on codes or categories that emerged from the data. I continue this step for the first four or five transcripts as these emerging categories are used to refine subsequent interview questions. My second step is to construct a table with columns to capture the emerging codes with a separate category labeled "other" to capture content that may appear to be an outlier or not a fit with the other emerging categories. I continue this process until all content from all interviews has found a home. My third step is to review the quotes inserted in each column and define each category. My fourth step is to review the definitions of each category and determine if any of the categories are similar enough to be collapsed. My goal is to never have more than 4–5 categories that I develop for any manuscript. If I am not able to collapse to a few categories, I then proceed to determine ways that I might separate the categories for additional manuscripts. A fifth step is to identify subcategories within each major category. Finally, in the construction of this coding table, I will have a column inserted to the far left with participant number and a brief description of this participant. Participant descriptions can be information collected from the demographic questionnaire as well as any information collected during observations recorded as field notes.

African American Women Breast Cancer Survivors: Coping with the COVID-19 Pandemic

Table 10.1 displays the category headings from a first draft of coding the data from the African American Women Breast Cancer Survivors Coping with COVID study (Hamilton et al., 2022). The study focused on coping during the COVID pandemic. The categories capture the content that emerged from the interview questions and probing. Participants generally talked about their perceptions of COVID as a life-threatening situation, the stressors experienced during the COVID pandemic, and their strategies for coping during the COVID pandemic. As you can see, this initial coding table had a column labeled *Other*, to house quotes where I was not sure where to place them.

In this second draft (see Table 10.2), I was able to refine the categories to be more specific with category labeling. For example, stressors were related to being isolated, disruptions in health care/appointments, and the overwhelming news from television and social

Table 10.1 First Draft of Coding Table

#	Stressors During Breast Cancer During Diagnosis	Stressors as Long-Term Survivor	Perceptions About COVID	Songs/Bible Verses to Cope	Other/Not Sure Where It Goes

Table 10.2 Second Draft of Coding Table

#	Isolated/Restricted Social Activities/ Being Vulnerable	Change in Health Care/Delays in Appointments/ Delays in Preventative Care	Source of COVID Information/ Seriousness	Follow the Rules	Other Changed to Types of Coping Family Support Religious Participation

media that COVID was a deadly illness. In this draft, I began to conceptualize religious songs and reading the Bible as types of religious practices that functioned similarly to content in the *Other* (family support) category as types of coping. As a result, these two categories were combined and relabeled.

In Table 10.3, I paired initial categories with exemplar quotes. In selecting exemplar quotes, I identify those that capture a complete thought and best illustrate the

Table 10.3 Exemplary Quotes (Draft)

Draft categories	*Exemplary quotes*
Isolated/ restricted social activities/being vulnerable	1 "And so I'm very active in my church so therefore I miss my church family. I miss the times that we get to come together on Sunday or on Wednesday evening or simply for just a meal. Not that we're not doing things online but it's different when we can't hug and greet each other. And yes I am a very sociable woman but I'm not stressed out to the fact to where I'm going to lose it if I don't have some type of social things going on"—Participant 1 2 "When I heard about that and the different health causes and stuff that are very receptive to it, your immune system and everything of course going through what I've gone through with chemo, radiation - all of that I definitely was like okay trying to be as safe as possible. Wearing my mask, my gloves. I don't want to go out unless it's to the store. I try to definitely do the distancing. I try to, well within my family we promote it."—Participant 14 3 "But corona - it's kind of stressful for you to be in the house all day long. It's very stressful."—Participant 7
Change in health care/ delays in appointments/ delays in preventative care:	1 My rheumatologist she had to give me a three-month supply of my Proximal because that is the drug they are using to treat Covid19. As I've been, you know, reading some of what my friends have on Facebook about having to go to the drugstore, you know, and they cannot get their medication because they are out. I'm in a panic, you know?" -Participant 9 2 "I'm a people person. I like to talk. I like to hug. So you know you have to change your whole outlook on life. And then whether to go to these appointments. Because I'm supposed to be going to an appointment to see my oncologist the twenty-eighth of this month but I called them and asked them if I could put it off for a month because I'm afraid to go to the hospital. I've got to have a PET scan and lab work and all of that. And then you know last January and February I was in the hospital. I'm going for infusions every eight weeks. My next infusion is due May the fifth. Do I go for my infusion? I'm still stumbling a little but I'm walking pretty good. I walk without my cane. Just trying to make safe decisions."—Participant 13 3 "The, the thing that bothers me every– like, at the end of the month, since we had this pandemic, I usually go every May to have the mammogram done. Well, I couldn't do this time; Emory closed. So, couldn't go, and then finally they sent a letter in the mail that, you know, they're open again and to schedule your appointment."—Participant 18

(*Continued*)

Table 10.3 (Continued)

Draft categories	*Exemplary quotes*
Source of COVID information/ seriousness	1 "I learned about it like everybody else did, on TV. And then when it came to be as bad as it is, my primary care physician she was on me like X make sure that you wash your hands every chance you get. Make sure that you wear your mask wherever you go because my immune system is double compromised now, you know? So I have to be extra cautious on even if I'm going out to the store to get my essentials."—Participant 9 2 "Just pretty much TV. Social media. Just watching the news and I watch the news all the time, all the time, all the time and then I had to stop, you know? I limit my portals of what's coming in because I was consumed with it because I was in fear. And it seems like I was more scared of this than I was of breast cancer. Why is the virus more threatening than cancer: "Because you heard more about the deaths than the survival of it and I think that's what did it? You know with breast cancer you hear about survivors. I'm a survivor. You hear about everybody who survived. So that made you feel like okay I can survive too. In the beginning with this pandemic they just made you focus on who was dying. Then you think about the bodies and seeing all that on TV it just seemed like it was more publicized than cancer - even though cancer you hear about it a lot. But it just focused more on the deaths. And then the fact that it was spreading from country to country like waves. So it just seemed like it put more fear because there's no cure. Even though there's no cure for the cancer but you know you can get treatments and that type of thing. With the pandemic what are the treatments? There are none. You have to just wait it out, you know? So that's what made it fearful."—Participant 10
Follow the rules	1 "We did go get the gloves - well I had gloves here. But we went and bought masks and more gloves. And we go out. When it first started you know, we would go to the grocery store without the mask and everything. But when it got worse that's when we started doing the gloves and the mask and everything."—Participant 6 2 "And I'm definitely not allowing this Coronavirus to stop me, you know from doing anything. I'm using wisdom and I'm using common sense. But I'm not going to stop living. I'm not. I'm not."—Participant 8 3 "My son has been going to get groceries. Mama you don't need to go anywhere. You're too old. So that's stressful. I like to look at my bananas. I don't want them too green. I don't want them too yellow. I want them straight. Then they send you substitutes if they don't have what you want. I wanted pineapple juice and they sent me grape juice. Grape juice got too much sugar in it."—Participant 13
Coping with songs/Bible verses/church and family support	1 "I just had a moment to where it's almost like fear tried to grip my heart. But I had to go inside and rely on what I knew to be true concerning the word of God. And for a moment there you know that's what I had to do. Well when you are a believer you're just that. You come to believe that even though you are here in this world you believe that God is greater than what you see around you. He's able to comfort you. He can protect you because his word says it and you become a believer in him. You become a believer in what he said. And that's my protection right there. That's the whole of who I am as a child of God with my faith. That's the whole of who I am. My faith is in God. Because if it wasn't I probably could only imagine what some people are actually experiencing today with everything that is going on. There's a lot of fear. There's a lot of anxiety. There is a lot of stress. There's a lot of hopelessness all around me. But I have learned enough."—Participant 1

(*Continued*)

Table 10.3 (Continued)

Draft categories	*Exemplary quotes*
	2 "My communication is not as prevalent as it was and that kind of gets me down sometimes because of this. Not able to go out and socialize. They do call and check on me and see how I'm doing. But I'm a hugger. I like to hug and I like to socialize. That has been taken. It's one thing if you don't go out because it's your choice. It's another thing when you don't have a choice or say in the matter. It kind of gets me down sometimes. And I've had some little emotional bouts in my home being by myself. I talk to God a lot. I have to, you know? That keeps me going. I talk to my family every day. We're on the phone every day. We can even do video chats and it's so nice. On Saturday Sisters Network got together and we did a Zoom."—Participant 8

category. I also select exemplar quotes that capture diverse voices, i.e., gender, age, educational level, or marital status. This table saves time and the work of returning to transcripts for exemplar quotes when disseminating the findings in oral presentations or manuscripts.

In Table 10.4, I illustrate the final labeling of categories and subcategories from the previous table. Similar categories were combined into subcategories to form a major category and given a label that captured a common theme among the subcategories. Note that the major categories capture the research questions: (1) what were the stressors experienced during COVID-19? and (2) what were the responses to the stressors during COVID-19?

Table 10.5 displays major categories, subcategories, definitions with exemplar quotes. This table is extremely helpful during manuscript writing, providing content needed for the findings section.

In my research, I have primarily used the process of content analysis since that is the method I learned in my doctoral studies. However, I could have easily used thematic analysis in any of the qualitative studies I have conducted. In the next section, I offer a summary of thematic analysis with a hypothetical example.

Thematic Analysis

The process of thematic analysis detailed by Braun and Clarke (2014) has been described in detail elsewhere and summarized in this section (Braun & Clarke, 2014). According to Braun and Clarke (2014), Thematic Analysis is an active process of identifying and selecting patterns of interest in the data and then reporting those identified themes to the reader. Although presented as a distinct method to analyze qualitative data, thematic analysis can be used in conjunction with qualitative research using grounded theory or qualitative descriptive approaches. That is, this method is useful regardless of whether or not a theoretical framework is used. However, should a theoretical framework be used, it is important to acknowledge the scholar's positioning and values underlying that framework. Although I have generally used concept analysis, I could have used thematic analysis since this method is also appropriate for research that explores participant illness experiences and realities that shape meanings related to those experiences. I am especially drawn to the work of Braun and

Table 10.4 Final Coding Categories and Subcategories

Major categories	*First draft subcategories*	*Final subcategories*
Stressors experienced during COVID	Isolated/restricted social activities/being vulnerable: Fear of COVID exposure Being homebound Isolated from church activities, missing church family	Potential COVID-19 spreaders in their immediate environments; Closures and restricted access to social and faith-based activities;
	Change in health care/delays in appointments/delays in preventative care: Struggles for prescription refills Fear of contracting COVID during office visits Delays in follow-up care Postponed cancer screening	Disruptions to planned cancer prevention and control health care
	Source of COVID-19 information/ seriousness: News of COVID-19 solely through TV created fear of death, dying Communication of COVID-19 being terminal, no cure	Televised news broadcasts of COVID-19
Responses to stressors of COVID	Isolated/restricted social activities/being vulnerable: Self-isolation strategies that were separated from a COVID-19-imposed isolation (school, church, barber, beauty salon closures)	Seeking COVID-19 information
	Following the rules includes: Needing to wear gloves, masks Finding a new normal, can't stop everything Staying away from crowed places where increased chances of contracting COVID-19	Following the rules
	Coping with songs/Bible verses/church and family support Faith in God Support from family and friends Finding new ways to socialize with fellow church members	Seeking support from God, family, and friends.

Table 10.5 Category/Subcategories with Definitions and Exemplar Quotes

Major category	*Subcategory*	*Definition*
Stressors during COVID	Potential COVID-19 Spreaders in Immediate Environments	Participants described being especially vulnerable to contracting this virus that could prove deadly given their immunocompromised system. These women spoke of the stress they felt when encountering family members who were not as careful about adhering to COVID-19 guidelines. Adhering to guidelines while living in a household with family members who were frontline workers or in occupations where social distancing was a challenge was especially frightening for these women. Mrs. Howard, a 59-year-old married, two-year survivor of stage 2 breast cancer spoke of the threat of contracting COVID-19 from multiple factors including her family. *Because you know it's up in the air. This virus is so unknown that you know, we don't know what the effects are for people who have our own immune suppressed medications and not only that, my age and all this kind of stuff so I'm very stressed out. I have not been out of the house more than twice in two or three weeks. And when I do go out, I wear my mask or gloves and stuff. And I'm not even in contact with anybody that has gone out. I don't even do a lot of contact with my husband. My children. None of that. Because you know I just want to isolate myself. Because I don't want to be exposed. And that in itself—not getting out, not going around doing stuff—that's stressful in itself.*
	Closures and restricted access to social and faith-based activities	Disruptions to church services and other social activities were especially stressful to these women. For Mrs. Cone, a 75-year-old, widowed, and 19-year survivor of stage 2 breast cancer, attending church was a major place for socialization with friends. However, she was not able to attend church during the pandemic. She described her feelings: *And so, I'm very active in my church so therefore I miss my church family. I miss the times that we get to come together on Sunday or on Wednesday evening or simply for just a meal. Not that we're not doing things online but it's different when we can't hug and greet each other. And yes, I am a very sociable woman, but I'm not stressed out to the fact to where I'm going to lose it if I don't have some type of social things going on.*

(*Continued*)

Table 10.5 (Continued)

Major category	*Subcategory*	*Definition*
	Televised news broadcasts of COVID-19	Source of information on the virus that was primarily from televised news (TV and social media) and overwhelming Mrs. Cone, the 75-year-old, widowed, and 19-year survivor of stage 2 breast cancer compared the threat of the virus to that of breast cancer as much more serious and deadly. *.. . I watch the news all the time, all the time, all the time and then I had to stop, you know? I limit my portals of what's coming in because I was consumed with it, because I was in fear. And it seems like I was more scared of this than I was of breast cancer. Why is the virus more threatening than cancer. . . ? Because you heard more about the deaths than the survival of it and I think that's what did it? You know with breast cancer you hear about survivors. I'm a survivor. You hear about everybody who survived. So that made you feel like, okay, I can survive too. In the beginning with this pandemic, they just made you focus on who was dying. Then you think about the bodies and seeing all that on TV, it just seemed like it was more publicized than cancer - even though cancer you hear about it a lot. But it just focused more on the deaths. And then the fact that it was spreading from country to country like waves. So, it just seemed like it put more fear because there's no cure. Even though there's no cure for the cancer but you know you can get treatments and that type of thing. With the pandemic, what are the treatments? There are none. You have to just wait it out, you know? So that's what made it fearful.*
	Disruptions to planned appointments for cancer preventative and control health care	There were concerns related to accessing prescribed medications as well as making decisions of whether or not to attend routine cancer screenings, also included delayed treatments. Ms. Johnson is a 48-year-old single, eight-year breast cancer survivor who described her fears of not being able to get medications from the drugstore due to limited supplies: *My rheumatologist she had to give me a three-month supply of my Proximal because that is the drug they are using to treat Covid-19. As I've been, you know, reading some of what my friends have on Facebook about having to go to the drugstore, you know, and they cannot get their medication because they are out. I'm in a panic, you know?*

(*Continued*)

Table 10.5 (Continued)

Major category	*Subcategory*	*Definition*
Responses to COVID Stressors	Seeking COVID-19 information	Self-isolation was used as a method of protection from contracting the virus. In doing so, this prevented these African American women from gaining further information regarding the pandemic at culturally important gatherings with family, friends, and fellow church members. Instead, they relied heavily on television and social media platforms for pandemic information. However, Mrs. Johnson, the 48-year-old survivor of stage 2 breast cancer, did get information on preventive measures from her primary care physician: *I learned about it like everybody else did—on TV. And then when it came to be as bad as it is, my primary care physician she was on me like "[Mrs. Johnson] make sure that you wash your hands every chance you get.. . Make sure that you wear your mask wherever you go" because my immune system is double compromised now, you know? So, I have to be extra cautious on even if I'm going out to the store to get my essentials.*
	Following the rules	Wearing masks, wearing gloves, social distancing, and not going out unless absolutely necessary were the rules these participants lived by to prevent contracting COVID-19. Even though many of them were several years post-treatment, these African American breast cancer survivors were aware of their vulnerability and potentially immunocompromised status. Mrs. Gates, a 47-year-old married, five-year survivor of stage 1 breast cancer, spoke of the importance of following the guidelines for the safety of her entire family: *When I heard about that and the different health causes and stuff that are very receptive to it, your immune system and everything of course going through what I've gone through with chemo, radiation - all of that, I definitely was like okay trying to be as safe as possible. Wearing my mask, my gloves. I don't want to go out unless it's to the store. I try to definitely do the distancing. I try to; well within my family we promote it.*

(*Continued*)

Table 10.5 (Continued)

Major category	*Subcategory*	*Definition*
	Seeking support from family, church family, and friends	Participants attempted to remain connected to family, church family, and friends during this pandemic while maintaining the social distancing guidelines. Churches closed their doors, and this further limited the ability of these participants to connect with family and friends. Communication through social media and telephone became the alternative approach for maintaining social connections. Ms. Williams, a 62-year-old, widowed, and two-year survivor of stage 2 breast cancer described her experience with socializing with family and friends during the COVID-19 pandemic: *My communication is not as prevalent as it was, and that kind of gets me down sometimes because of this. Not able to go out and socialize. They [family and friends] do call and check on me and see how I'm doing. But I'm a hugger. I like to hug, and I like to socialize. That has been taken away. It's one thing if you don't go out because it's your choice. It's another thing when you don't have a choice or say in the matter. It kind of gets me down sometimes. And I've had some little emotional 'bouts in my home being by myself. I talk to God a lot. I have to, you know? That keeps me going. I talk to my family every day. We're on the phone every day. We can even do video chats and it's so nice. On Saturday we [support group] got together, and we did a Zoom.*

Clarke (2014) given their emphasis on explicitly stating the choices made during the research process. These scholars remind us that the product produced from our qualitative research is very much an active process that consists of a series of actions and choices. Moreover, this process is one that should capture the experience of participants guided by the research question(s) of an understudied topic among an understudied population.

Although not a theory, my research has generally been guided by a cultural equivalence perspective (Hamilton, 2001). According to this framework, it is important that scholars consider whether the use of any concepts, methods, or data captured from measures misrepresents a population. That is, comparisons of populations do not ignore the cultural context or cultural relevance of populations in the interpretation of findings. When concepts based solely on the lived experiences of a majority or dominant group are used as the standard for judging the behaviors of a minority group, researchers assume cultural equivalence (Marin & Marin, 1991). In addition, when conceptualizations of variables based on the lived experiences of the dominant Caucasian group are the norm by which behaviors of members of other racial and ethnic groups are judged, research findings distinguishing the behavior of the minority group are often found to be statistically nonsignificant. Moreover, in studies comparing Caucasians to minority groups, members of other racial or ethnic groups are often viewed as pathologic or deviant (Billingsley, 1988; Wilson, 1986). Research that routinely reveals the deficits of a population may also obscure the realities of what is meaningful to that population (Billingsley, 1992).

In healthcare research, cultural equivalence is seen when groups are compared using one of the groups as the standard for making judgments about both. Although healthcare researchers use race, gender, class, or some combination of these categories for the purpose of comparing differences in groups, the use of race, particularly black/white comparisons occur most frequently (Laveist et al., 1995). These black/white comparison studies that examine differences have typically used the lifestyles, attitudes, and health behaviors of white males as the standard or norm by which to judge other groups (Gamble, 1993).

Comparing various aspects of the African American lived experiences to those of Caucasians without consideration for cultural differences has resulted in negative evaluations, misinformation, and stereotypes (Collins, 1991; Gamble, 1993). Historically, medical research that compared African Americans to Caucasians supported assumptions of biological differences that justified societal attitudes and beliefs that African Americans were an inferior race (Gamble, 1993). Because of these comparisons, researchers in the late 19th and early 20th centuries supported the notion that African Americans were inferior in their anatomy, in control of their sexual desires, and morals (Gamble, 1993; Williams et al., 1994). In a review of those negative assumptions reported in medical and public health journals, Gamble (1993) found excessive reports of higher syphilis rates which were attributed to an excessive sexual desire and immorality they believed existed among African Americans. Given this perspective, I am always cognizant that the research I conduct captures the voices of African Americans in the most rigorous way possible and represents the strengths and weaknesses of the target population with minimal bias.

Quantitative Analysis

Although the main focus of qualitative data analysis has focused on text from transcribed interviews, I also conduct quantitative analysis using a statistical program. The use of a quantitative statistical program allows me to examine text quantitatively and construct tables for demographic data and counting of categories or themes for oral and written presentations. Quantitative analysis also permits me to explore statistical differences frequencies of categories using the Chi-square or Fisher's exact test. I have used these tests when conducting a qualitative project with large numbers of participants.

Tables 10.6 and 10.7 illustrate the use of Chi-square or Fisher's exact test to examine whether frequencies of demographic characteristics or stressful event were statistically significant among groups of participants. Table 10.6 shows statistically significant

Table 10.6 Demographics of Sample by Age Group

	Young old (50–64) *(n = 22)*	*Middle old (65–74)* *(n = 21)*	*Oldest old (≥75)* *(n = 22)*	*(F or X^2)*
Age				
Mean (*SD*)	56 (4.0)	68 (2.8)	82 (4.8)	$F = 241.05$**
Gender				
Male	3 (13.6%)	8 (38.1%)	8 (36.4%)	
Female	19 (86.4%)	13 (61.9%)	14 (63.6%)	$X^2 = 3.93$
Education				
Less than HS	2 (9.1%)	0 (0%)	11 (50%)	
Completed HS	5 (22.7%)	14 (66.7%)	8 (36.4%)	
Completed College	15 (68.2%)	7 (33.3%)	3 (13.6%)	$X^2 = 32.30$**
Marital status				
Married	12 (54.5%)	10 (47.6%)	9 (40.9%)	
Not married	10 (45.5%)	11 (52.4%)	13 (59.1%)	$X^2 = 21.90$*
Employment status				
Employed	14 (63.6%)	3 (14.3%)	0 (0%)	
Disabled	5 (22.7%)	3 (14.3%)	0 (0%)	
Retired	3 (13.6%)	15 (71.4%)	22 (100%)	$X^2 = 37.24$**
Religious affiliation *(Early years)*				
Baptist	16 (72.7%)	14 (66.7%)	15 (68.2%)	
Missionary Baptist	1 (4.5%)	1 (4.8%)	1 (4.5%)	
AME	2 (9.1%)	3 (14.3%)	3 (13.6%)	
AME Zion	1 (4.5%)	0 (0%)	1 (4.5%)	
Catholic	2 (9.1%)	3 (14.3%)	1 (4.5%)	
CME	0 (0%)	0 (0%)	1 (4.5%)	$X^2 = 4.36$
Religious affiliation *(Adult years)*				
Baptist	14 (63.6%)	16 (76.2%)	17 (77.3%)	
Missionary Baptist	0 (0%)	1 (4.8%)	1 (4.5%)	
AME	1 (4.5%)	1 (4.8%)	2 (9.1%)	
AME Zion	1 (4.5%)	0 (0%)	1 (4.5%)	
Catholic	4 (18.2%)	2 (9.2%)	1 (4.5%)	
Holiness	1 (4.5%)	2 (9.2%)	0 (0%)	$X^2 = 7.67$
Community size				
Rural	16 (72.7%)	12 (57.1%)	5 (22.7%)	
Urban	6 (27.3%)	9 (42.9%)	17 (77.3%)	$X^2 = 11.51$*

* $p \leq .05$
** $p \leq .01$

differences among participants according to age, gender, education, marital status, and geographical location.

Table 10.7 uses Chi-square or Fisher's exact test to examine differences in stressful event among age groups. A statistically significant difference occurred when the stressful event was the family death of a spouse among the oldest old group of participants.

Table 10.7 Stressful Event by Age Group

Event	*Young old (50–64)*	*Middle old (65–74)*	*Oldest old (≥75)*	X^2
	(n = 22)	*(n = 21)*	*(n = 22)*	
Family death event				
Spouse	2	2	11	13.58**
Mother	5	10	9	3.09
Father	8	6	5	.99
Child	2	2	3	.29
Sibling	5	5	3	.85
Illness event				
Cancer	11	7	5	3.64
Heart disease/CV	1	3	5	3.05
Trauma/accident	1	3	0	3.95
Other chronic illness	7	4	7	1.16
Work-related event	3	2	1	1.09

**$p \leq .01$

Note: Participants could have had more than one stressful event.

Conclusion

In this chapter on qualitative analysis strategies, I focus primarily on Content Analysis with examples from my research on SDOH and African American cancer patients. Additional content is provided on Thematic Analysis for the reader with a preference for this strategy. Important to note, however, is the necessity to explain the rationale for any approach used. My preference for Content Analysis was a result of what I was encouraged to use during my doctoral training. I end my career with the regret of never analyzing any of my data using narrative analysis to capture the way in which African American cancer patients told their survivorship stories from a place of strength and not weakness as is so often assumed.

References

Billingsley, A. (1988). *Black Families in White America*. New Jersey, Prentice-Hall.

Billingsley, A. (1992). *Climbing Jacob's Ladder: The Enduring Legacy of African-American Families*. New York, Simon & Schuster.

Braun, V. and V. Clarke. (2014). "What can "thematic analysis" offer health and wellbeing researchers?" *Int J Qual Stud Health Well-being* **9**: 26152.

Collins, P. H. (1991). *Black Feminist Thought*. New York, Routledge, Chapman and Hall.

Gamble, V. N. (1993). "A legacy of distrust: African Americans and medical research." *J Prev Medicine* **9**(6): 35–38.

Hamilton, J. (2001). *Theorizing social support among African Americans with cancer*. Doctoral Dissertation, Chapel Hill, NC, University of North Carolina.

Hamilton, J. B., N. C. Best, T. A. Barney, V. C. Worthy and N. R. Phillips (2022). "Using spirituality to cope with COVID-19: The experiences of African American Breast Cancer Survivors." *J Cancer Educ* **37**(5): 1422–1428. doi: 10.1007/s13187-021-01974-8

Hsieh, H. F. and S. E. Shannon. (2005). "Three approaches to qualitative content analysis." *Qual Health Res* **15**(9): 1277–1288.

Laveist, T. A., J. M. Wallace and D. L. Howard. (1995). "The color line and the health of African Americans." *Humboldt J Soc Relati* **21**: 119–137.

Marin, G. and B. V. Marin. (1991). *Research With Hispanic Populations*. Newbury Park, CA, Sage Publications.

Sandelowski, M. (2010). "What's in a name? Qualitative description revisited." *Res Nurs Health* **33**(1): 77–84.

Strauss, A. and J. Corbin. (1998). *Basics of Qualitative Research: Techniques and Procedures for Developing Grounded Theory*. Thousand Oaks, CA, Sage.

Williams, D. R., R. Lavizzo-Mourey and R. C. Warren. (1994). "The concept of race and health status in America." *Public Health Rep* **109**(1): 26–41.

Wilson, M. N. (1986). "The Black extended family: An analytical consideration." *Dev Psychol* **22**(2): 246–258. doi: 10.1037/0012-1649.22.2.246

11 Success in the Academy as a Qualitative Researcher

I have had a wonderful career in the academy as a qualitative researcher and tenured professor in a research-intensive school of nursing. In this chapter, I discuss the five general areas that contributed to this success. These areas are rigorous research training with internationally renowned scientists, a passion that drives meaningful research questions, the ability to secure funding to support the research, and most importantly, the skills and knowledge to disseminate the research in peer-reviewed journals.

Research Training and Mentorship

In my doctoral studies, I had the privilege to learn concepts related to qualitative methods and analysis with Dr. Margarete Sandelowski, an internationally known qualitative research scholar. While the coursework provided a strong foundation for the conduct of qualitative research, the critical contributing factor for my success was the additional research training and mentoring that I received beyond the classroom instruction. I have been especially privileged to have decades of mentorship and research training with Dr. Sandelowski who served as Chair of my dissertation research, *Theorizing Social Support among African American Cancer Patients*. After graduating from the University of North Carolina at Chapel Hill with my PhD, Dr. Sandelowski continued in her role as research mentor by assisting me with manuscript writing. This partnership resulted in two first-authored papers from my dissertation research. During my early and mid-career years as faculty, Dr. Sandelowski continued mentoring me, guiding my development of advanced qualitative methods and strengthening the skills that enabled me to educate and train emerging qualitative researchers.

It is also important to mention that it is vital to seek out mentors that share your vision and passion for the research questions that drive your research. During my PhD program when presenting my work at research conferences, I would encounter PhD students from other nursing schools who commented that they wanted to conduct projects with similar research questions but were not permitted to do so. I realize now that my training also included encouragement to pursue research questions that would permit me to explore the strengths of a population and not just its weaknesses or that which was lacking. Dr. Sandelowski once told me not to follow in her footsteps but to find my own way. It was years before I understood this directive, which I greatly appreciate now. During your training as an SDOH Qualitative Researcher, remember to include interdisciplinary scholars who are experts with your specific population. These individuals may be content experts in a disease or illness, experts in the culture, or experts in the history of the target population. Throughout my career, I have sought out the mentorship of a number of individuals

DOI: 10.4324/9781003598916-11

including that of a community member and African American cancer survivor with whom I have had a close collaborative relationship for many years.

The years of research training, mentorship, and finding my own way have resulted in this textbook, *Using Qualitative Methods for Social Determinants of Health Research.* I am hopeful that the content of this text will facilitate the user's application of qualitative methods in SDOH research in the health sciences and that it will provide a source of information and instruction not readily available in my earlier years as an emerging nurse scientist.

Qualitative Methods to Drive Meaningful Research

Throughout my career, the NIH funding I received as PI to support my research has been for quantitative studies (measurement, intervention pilot work). As an Assistant Professor, I was the recipient of extramural funding (NIH/NCI P60 pilot study, NIH/NINR/NCMHD R01) that permitted me to survive in an academic environment that measured success primarily through the acquisition of NIH funding. This NIH funding was critical for my survival in the academic environment during those days and facilitated my success in transitioning from Assistant Professor to tenured Associate Professor. However, the research that has been most meaningful in my career has been from explorations of phenomena using qualitative research. I have often reflected on the reasons for a preference for research questions that required qualitative methods. The likely reason for this desire for qualitative methods reflects my desire to conduct the work that is not only meaningful to me but to the population responsible for my achievements as a nurse scientist. I frequently tell the story of the encounter with a former nursing faculty who once made the comment that the only truths about a population were those that made it to peer-reviewed journals. This faculty was specifically referring to a few studies that concluded that African Americans experiencing chronic illness lacked social support. I rejected that thinking, especially given the ways I saw older African Americans support each other during illness and bereavement. While I did not know at the time why those negative conclusions were drawn, I became committed to changing that narrative. Since that time, I have made it my mission to capture and publish a different truth about the health and well-being of African American populations. This different truth comes from the voices of African Americans who are fortunate enough to have scientists capture and disseminate their stories. During my time in the academy, I have attempted to represent a truth that African Americans are not always deviant or pathologic, but have experiences that have enabled them to survive for generations. Specifically, my program of research has focused on promoting optimal coping strategies among older African Americans during encounters with life-threatening illness. The research questions that have emerged from the information were transmitted to me from the stories that captured the experiences of underrepresented populations in underserved communities.

Funding Qualitative Research

A major concern for scientists in the academy is securing funding to conduct their research. For scientists in health care at research-intensive universities, the benchmark is generally extramural funding from the National Institutes of Health. However, projects designed to answer research questions designed solely for the use of qualitative methods are likely to not appeal to reviewers on NIH study sections or to be consistent with funding priorities of NIH Institutes. While the NIH and its institutes may focus on quantitative, population-level studies, there is still significant room for qualitative projects that not only enrich quantitative studies but also build and corroborate knowledge in their own right. It is important to remember that common themes in university mission statements include academic excellence, the creation and application of knowledge, and to promote a culture of humanity to improve the human condition.

Throughout my career, I have successfully conducted meaningful SDOH research using qualitative methods without NIH funding. The primary cost of conducting qualitative research projects is the time commitment. I have been able to support several qualitative studies with discretionary funds negotiated with school leadership, as well as from indirect costs associated with NIH-funded studies. The actual cost of conducting a qualitative research project with a sample size of 20–30 participants can be relatively low, requiring gift cards and funds to pay for the transcribing of interviews or focus groups. The cost of time comes from conducting the interviews, especially if travel to participant homes is required. Often, I have not taken the time to seek funding for the qualitative work since this process (drafting the proposal, waiting for the review, resubmission of the proposal) would delay moving my research forward. My process was to always conduct the qualitative research, submit the quantitative proposal, analyze and disseminate the qualitative research, then revise and resubmit the quantitative proposal. This process permitted me to keep proposals under review but also maintain a continuous record of disseminating data-based manuscripts.

Publishing Qualitative Research

Success in the academy seems to be equated with the acquisition of research dollars; however, I have always argued that the real benchmark for success is dissemination of knowledge. The primary goal of any scientist should be to publish and publish often. During my predoctoral and postdoctoral studies, I received a number of NIH training grants—my time as an emerging scientist was filled with moving from one study to the next. I was not only conducting my own research, but as a recipient of predoctoral research training fellowships, I was engaged in my mentors' research activities as well. This pattern of seeking funding and conducting research projects continued well into my role as Assistant Professor. I had secured a number of intramural and extramural research awards but most importantly, I had received the NIH R01 Award within three years of completing my postdoctoral studies. I was a success in the academy, or so I thought.

Early in my career as an Assistant Professor, I definitely met the criteria for excellence in securing research grants for quantitative studies, but after four years as Assistant Professor on tenure track, I only had four publications. During my predoctoral studies, I was a research assistant on NIH studies and learned to collect data, conduct focus groups, and deliver interventions, but had not been included on publications. The four publications from my dissertation research were nowhere near what was needed for me to successfully advance to Associate Professor. I knew I needed more publications. I examined the CVs of other recently promoted Assistant Professors in research-intensive environments who had 14–20 publications. Yet, the advice I received for transitioning to Associate Professor was to secure another NIH R01 Award. I tell this story because I am frequently contacted by predoctoral students, postdoctoral fellows, and Assistant and Associate Professors for advice on seeking faculty positions or promotion to Associate or Full Professor. Oftentimes, these individuals are in the same position as I was. They spend lots of effort writing proposals and conducting studies but very little on publications. These individuals are faced with "catching up" and writing feverishly to meet some publishing metric to secure that first job as Assistant Professor or to meet that metric for promotion. It was seven years after my postdoctoral fellowship that I figured out the publishing game and what "publish or perish" really means in the academy. In fact, I remember to this day being on the phone with my mentor who told me that my goal should be to publish five papers every year. I remember thinking, how in the world am I going to do that? I remember not being in a good place with my program of research. I had completed a measurement R01 and disseminated the findings from that research project. However, while I had been successful with NIH funding as an early-stage investigator, my subsequent NIH proposals were competing with senior researchers and proposals submitted by research teams. I was *dead in the water*.

Once I completed the call with my mentor and stopped hyperventilating at the thought of needing five publications a year, I developed a plan. I didn't have a research team or colleagues to write with. I had been asked to participate in other research teams, but my requested role was to serve as a consultant or to collect data from an African American population. Not PI, not MPI, which are the roles needed to show independence in research scholarship for promotion. The primary requests for my contribution to research projects were to help collect the data. I would be paid well, but not included in dissemination of findings.

I knew that I needed publications. I refused to give up. I had seen other faculty not survive the academy for lack of productivity with publications. Some would argue that productivity includes success with grant awards, but the two go hand-in-hand. Publications are needed for success with grant awards, and grant awards are needed to produce data for success with publishing. Rather than focus on what I did not have, I focused on my strengths. I had the skill set to conduct qualitative research and I had discretionary funds for gift cards for incentives for participants. Although colleagues had no interest in my research questions, I had student mentees who also needed publications. I had been in regular contact with my very first research assistant who was in a master's program. We both needed publications, me for promotion and her for a PhD. I was privileged to be introduced to a clinical faculty member who needed publications for promotion on her track. A third contact was a community leader, cancer survivor, and registered nurse who requested mentoring to obtain a master's degree in nursing. The fourth individual was a recent PhD student needing assistance to publish his dissertation. These individuals became my initial research team. Over the years, students and faculty of all ranks have contributed to my list of publications. I am grateful for the contribution of their knowledge and skills to my success. and hopefully, I have contributed to their success.

Throughout this book, I have described the qualitative research projects I led over the years so I will not repeat descriptions of these again. I will describe how I, with my mentees, was successful with disseminating findings from qualitative research. The research team is important but strategies to maneuver the process of publishing in high impact peer-reviewed journals are critical. I am grateful to a former mentor and Department Chair, Dr. Marilyn Oermann, for teaching me strategies for publishing that enabled my survival in the academy. I present these strategies in the section to follow.

The first publishing strategy is to select three journals that publish qualitative research using similar formatting. In the selection of these journals, I consider the author requirements but criteria such as sample size and topics of interest. Even when the journal publishes qualitative reports, the editorial teams are likely to review through a quantitative lens.

Reviewers may selectively emphasize or ignore principles of qualitative research and base their acceptance or rejection of a manuscript on rigid principles that are not relevant to the research conducted. For example, reviewers will frequently require a sample size of 20–30 participants even though the sample size of qualitative reports should be based on saturation. A second principle that may lead a reviewer to reject a qualitative manuscript is a requirement for member checking with participants that occurs after data collection, ignoring variations in the application of this principle with underserved populations (see Chapter 8). Finally, reviewers in healthcare journals are likely to reject qualitative manuscripts if the data is more than five years old. Is there nothing to be learned from participant stories or experiences older than five years? Stories older than five years are not discarded in History, Anthropology, and English. Why do we not value the relevance of these stories in health care?

A second reason to select three journals for your manuscript submission that are similarly formatted is simple. If the editorial review rejects the manuscript as not being a fit for their journal, you are prepared to send it right back out to another journal. Do not edit or second guess the quality of the manuscript. Accept that the manuscript wasn't a good fit or the editor may have a manuscript in the pipeline similar to yours. Hopefully, this initial rejection occurs after a couple of weeks so you are able to resubmit quickly. Whatever you do, do not give up. You may have to submit and resubmit, revise and revise again. Many of the published qualitative papers you are reading were submitted to more than one journal and were required to respond to reviewer critiques more than once. Responding to reviewer criticism is hard, but oftentimes reviewers' comments really do improve the manuscript. You may, however, need to reach out to the editor for assistance with overly critical reviews. Be persistent, your manuscript will find a home.

The second publishing strategy is to form a research team or writing collaborators. If you are not able to establish a team or find collaborators in your immediate environment, look for individuals from other departments or even other universities. Given advances in technology and our ability to communicate globally, there is no need to be restricted with whom you will collaborate. Be creative. You may be turned down, but you will eventually find partners who share your vision and are eager to work with you. In this process, you will come across individuals who lack integrity and are just not responsible. You will encounter these individuals throughout your career but don't let them distract you. Give firm deadlines and excuse these individuals from your writing team. If the individual is a person of power at your institution, continue with the manuscript, submit, and move on. You do not have to continue to publish with them.

In forming your research team for publishing, remember that your team of researchers does not have to look like what you saw in your predoctoral or postdoctoral program. Consider colleagues at other institutions, colleagues you meet at research conferences, and clinical faculty at your institution. Even emerging scientists that are currently undergraduate and graduate students at your institution will welcome the opportunity to learn from you and use this experience to support their transition to the next phase of their careers. I always emphasize the need to include members of the community and target populations in the dissemination of findings. These individuals may not have the training of scientists, but are a critical component of developing research questions that are relevant to the population. Community and members of the target population can provide valuable insight into the research project to ensure a more accurate representation of findings and conclusions drawn. The two manuscripts I had accepted without revisions as well as those with minimal revisions had the input of a community collaborator.

A final publishing strategy is to have a strong support system. The work to survive the metrics for success in the academy is stressful. Having support to discuss the challenges you will encounter during the submissions and rejections of manuscripts is crucial. Be sure to have lifelong mentors. Find mentors who share and understand your cultural background, who share your passion for the work you are doing, and who understand the demands of the academy. These mentors will cheer you on, provide honest critique, and much needed career advice. Also consider that learning is reciprocal. I have learned a great deal from my mentees over the years and increasingly rely on them for their feedback. One of the pleasures of my career has been watching my mentees grow professionally and to now learn from them.

Conclusion

The key to success in the academy for any scientist is mentoring and persistence. As a qualitative researcher, you are likely to encounter limited access to research training from senior faculty experienced in this methodology. You may also experience funding droughts for this research methodology and challenges with publishing in high-impact, peer-reviewed journals. Despite these challenges, it is possible to have a highly productive and rewarding career using qualitative methods particularly when the topic is SDOH. Mentoring from a diverse group of scholars who provide training in qualitative methods as well as scholars who are content experts is critical. I was fortunate to have had mentoring throughout my career and to continue to have mentoring as a senior, tenured faculty member. Although time-consuming, qualitative research can be conducted when finances are strained, and therefore suitable to collect data for publication when data from larger quantitative studies may be delayed. For me, the use of qualitative methods has supported a career of SDOH research highlighted by meaningful research questions and findings. In addition, my research has informed the work of other scientists, and it has broadened what we know about SDOH relative to underserved populations.

Index

Note: **Bold** pages refer to tables.